HANDBOOK
on
PARASITOLOGY

HANDBOOK
on
PARASITOLOGY

K. RENUKA

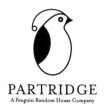

PARTRIDGE

A Penguin Random House Company

To order additional copies of this book, contact
Partridge India
000 800 10062 62
orders.india@partridgepublishing.com

www.partridgepublishing.com/india

CONTENTS

UNIT – I

INTRODUCTION

I Parasitology

A branch of Biology which deals with the inter – relationship between intraspecific animals or individuals (two animals) is called as parasitology. For better understanding of parasitology, we have to understand the different between Parasite, Parasitism and Parasitology

a) Parasite. is an animal which depends on other animals for their life processes.
b) Parasitism is an act of living on other animal.
c) Parasitology is the study of inter-relationship between two individuals.

Parasitology is an important branch of science where in we deal with basic questions like:

1. Why an animal depends on other animal, how and where aspects have to be studied.
2. It deals with human diseases and causes for the diseases.
3. Study of variety of relationship of parasites and their life cycle, hosts, influence on host, mode of transfer.

    i.   Etiology (an organism which is responsible for causing a disease).
    ii.   Prevalence (area of distribution)
    iii. Epidemiology (study of distribution and existence of organism in particular geographical area)

iv. Pathogenesis (study with deals with the pathogenic or pathological conditions caused by parasite).

v. Symptomology (symptoms of the disease)

vi. Diagnosis (clinical test)

vii. Immunology

viii. Prevention and control

II. Importance of Parasitology

Parasitology is studied by Parasitologist, Biochemists, Physiologists, Chemotheraphtic, Morphologists, Ecologists, Ethologists and Epidemiologists.

Parasitology is novel route finder of Physiological adaptations, Biochemical adaptations, Morphological adaptations and Wide range of immunity

III. What is parasitism?

For clear understanding of the concept parasitism, it is necessary to understand different types of associations and they are:

Symbiosis: Symbiosis comes from the Greek word symboiown (= to leave together). The term symbiosis could broadly be used to include all the different kinds of relationship which exist in nature.

A. Phoresis:

This term is used for a particular type of association in which one organism (larger) merely provides shelter, support or transport for another (smaller) organism of a different species

Ex: Fishes belonging to the genus *Fierashfris* which live within the respiratory tract of Holothurians or occasionally starfish. These fishes are relatively helpless and are readily attacked and discovered by other species; therefore they seek the transport from holothurians, which appears to be undistributed by the presence of the fish.

In Phoresis there is no metabolic dependence of either of the associates on the other. This type of phenomenon could clearly represent a stage similar to that in the early evolution of parasitism, since chance contact followed by the use of one species and shelter by the other is likely to have been the first step in an association leading to the parasitic way of life.

B. Commensalism:

The term literary means 'eating at the same table'. It is a type of loose association between animals of different species is which two animals live together without either being metabolically dependent on the other, although one or both organism may receive some benefit from the association. It is more important to stress, the absence of metabolic dependence in this type of association, for it is the absence of this feature, in particularly which separates a commensal sharply from a parasite. This association is not intimate since the tissue of the commensals is not in organic contact nor need it be permanent.

Ex: 1. Hermit crab (*Eupaguerus prideauxi*) and Sea anemone. Certain species of hermit crab and sea – anemones, in which the anemone lives on the shell sheltering access to the food caught and scattered or unwanted by the crab, whereas the crab benefits by the presence of the sea – anemone which assists in warding off undesirable predators. The crab crawls into shell which is too small for itself and uses the pedal disc of the anemone as cover for the unprotected position of its body (Ex: endocommensalism,).

2. Oxpicker Birds and African Mammals: The birds feed on the lice and ticks of mammals such as rhinoceroses and server to warn them of approaching enemy by displaying their own independent reactions. (Ex: ectocommensalism)

C. Parasitism

Of all the types of animal associations, perhaps parasitism has been, in the past, the most difficult to define. This has been largely due to the failure to recognize that the term has only a relative meaning but also to the insistence, by most authors, that a parasite must necessarily be harmful to its host animals.

To be classified as a parasite an organism must not only be in continuous intimate association with an individual of a different species, but it must also be metabolically dependent on it to some degree.

At one end of the hypothetical scale, is zero dependence, i.e. a free – living organisms; at the other end is 100 percent dependence or total parasitism. In between these two extremes are a range of organisms which satisfy their metabolic requirements to a varying extent at the expense of the host.

Diagram showing the relative concept of parasitism based on the degree of metabolic dependence: (a free living organism shows 0% dependence; a Cestode shows virtually 100% dependence. All degrees between these two extremes are encountered)

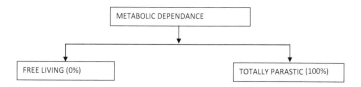

Although at first sight it would appear that most parasites are only dependent on their hosts for food materials, a closes examination shows that the situation is more complex than this. The parasite may be dependent on the host for one or more of the following:

   a.   Developmental stimuli
   b.   Nutritional material
   c.   Digestive enzymes
   d.   Control of maturation.

Parasite is unilaterally, metabolically, obligatorily and depends on host either permanently, sporadically, temporarily or periodically. To have a successful parasitic life, the following are most important: Communicable (of the parasite); well being of the host; temperature of the host and nutrition as provided by the host.

Presence of parasites may be known by:

i.   Disease:

   a.   Clinical stage (Treatment necessary)
   b.   Subclinical stage (Parasite don't cause more harm and pain is not felt)

      Condition of infected individual is impaired (not normal)

ii.   Infection: It is a process in with a parasite enters, establishes and multiplies in host.
iii. Pathogenicity and virulence: Organism's ability to cause disease in host.
iv.   Susceptibility Suspect (likelihood) of the host acquiring infection.
v.   Resistance: Defense mechanism of the host body in response to infection.
vi.   Immunity: Host's ability to resist specific infection.

D. Mutualism

It is a symbiotic association in which mutualist (small organism which is undergoing symbiotic relation with larger animal) and host are mutually, obligatory and metabolically dependent upon each other.

Ex: 1. Lichens: Fungi + Algae (Fungi help in absorption of water and Algae helps in photosynthesis).

   2. In the gut of wood eating termites, *Hypermastigote* flagellate are present. The termites eat wood but they do not posses cellulose enzyme with is substituted by the flagellate with secret or synthesis cellulose to digest cellulose. If they are separated then both termites and flagellate die.

UNIT – II

PATHOGENESIC
MICRO–ORGANISM

I. Brief classification of pathogenic bacteria:

The process of identification and devising the pathogens in appropriate way and arrangement, cataloging and using binomial nomenclature devised by Linnaeus is referred as classification.

II. Types of classification:

There are two ways of classifying bacteria, they are

1. Phylogenetic classification (for animals)
2. Adensomia or Numerical or score type of classification, based on number of characters resembling other organism (morphological features, biochemical features and physiological features).

In 1923 Bergys wrote: Manual of determinative Bacteriology 19 Vernacular names:

I. Photosynthetic bacteria (many bacteria)
II. Gliding bacteria (Movement based)
III. Sheathed bacteria (Sheath cover based)
IV. Budding and / or appendage bacteria
V. Spirochactes / spiral shaped body)
VI. Spirales and curved bacteria
VII. Gram –ve aerobic (rods and cocci)
VIII. Gram –ve facultative anaerobic (rods)
IX. Gram –ve anaerobic bacteria
X. Gram –ve (cocci and cocobacilli)
XI. Gram –ve anaerobic (cocci)

XII.   Gram –ve chemolithotrophic bacteria

XIII.   Methane producing bacteria

XIV.   Gram + ve cocci

XV.   Endospore forming rods and cocci

XVI.   Gram +ve Asporogenous (rods shaped bacteria)

XVII.   Actinomycetes and related organism

XVIII. Rickettrias

XIX.   Mycoplasmas.

1. Based on staining property bacteria can be classified as

    i.   Gram +Ve

    ii. Gram –ve (Pathogenic nature)

2. Based on shape

    i.   Rod shaped bacteria

    ii.   Round shaped bacteria

    iii. Spiral shaped bacteria

    iv.   Comma shaped bacteria

    v.   Diplococci / two held together

3. Based on filtration: filterable and non-filterable

Sterilization

Sterilization is defined as the process by which an article surface or medium is freed of all micro-organisms either in vegetative or spore state; disinfection means the destruction or all pathogenic bacteria (organism). The term antiseptic is used to indicate the prevention of the infection usually by inhibiting the growth of the bacteria. Bactericidal agents are those which are able to kill bacteria. Bacteriostatic agents only prevent the multiplication of bacteria and they may remain active. The various agents used in sterilization can be classified as follows:

Methods of Sterilization

A. Removal of microbes by lethal agents

i. Sterilization by heat: Heat is the most reliable methods of sterilization. Materials damageable by heat can be sterilized at lower temperature for longer periods or by repeated cycles. The factors influencing the sterilization by heat are:

1. Nature of heat whether dry heat or moist heat
2. Temperature and time
3. The number of micro organism.
4. The characteristic of the organism such as species, strain, sporing capacity.
5. The type of material from which the organism have to be eradicated.

The mechanism by which organism are destroyed by moist heat is different from that of the dry heat. The killing affect of the micro-organisms by dry heat is due to the denaturation of protein. Oxidative damage and the toxic affect are elevated at the levels of electrolytes. The lethal affect of the moist heat is due to the denatured and coagulation of the protein. In the case of spore steam condenses on it, increases its water content which ultimate hydrolysis and breakdown the bacterial protein. In complete moisture free atmosphere bacteria like many protein are more resistant to heat. They are killed when oxidation of the cell constituent occur. This requires much higher temperature than that needed for coagulation of protein.

The time required for sterilization is inversely proportional to the temperature of exposure. This can be expressed as thermal death time in which minimum time is required to kill a suspension of organism at a predetermined temperature in a specified investigation. The sterilization time is directly related to number of microbes in the suspension sterilization by heat is carried by 2 methods mainly.

a.   Dry heart
b.   Wet (Moist) heat

a. Dry heat

Hot air oven: This is the most widely used method of sterilization by dry heat. A holding period of 160°C for one hour is used to sterilize the glass ware, forceps, scissor all glass syringe some pharmaceutical products such as liquid paraffin's, sulphnamide diluting powder greases stress.

Hot air is a good conductor of heat and its penetrating power is low, the oven is usually heated electrically. The material in oven is arranged in such a manner that which allows free circulation of air in between all the glass wares for perfectly drying and should be plugged with cotton wool other glass waves such as petriplates etc should be wrapped in Kraft paper (Aluminum foils). After the complete process of heating, the oven should be cooled slowly for about two hours or else the glass ware may be cracked by sudden / uneven cooling. But this method is applicable to only heat resisting objects where as the liquid material cannot be used by this method as liquids evaporate.

b Wet (Moist) heat: (Using auto calve)

The principal of autoclave / steam sterilizer is that water boils where its vapors pressure equals to that of the surrounding atmosphere pressure. Hence when pressure inside a closed vessel increases the temperature at which water boils also increases. Saturated steam has greater penetrative power.

Sterilization by steam under pressure is carried out at temperature between 108°C and 147°C, thus using the appropriate temperature and time a variety of material such as dressing instruments, laboratory ware and pharmaceutical product can be sterilized, aqueous solution are sterilized between 108°C and 126°C several types of steam sterilization are in use:

1. Laboratory autoclave
2. Hospital autoclave
3. Bowel and instruments sterilization and
4. Rapid cooling sterilizers

B. Sterilization by chemicals

We have a wide range of chemical agents used as antiseptic and disinfectant remarkably little is known about the mechanism of action of many of these agents.

a. Alcohols

Ethyl alcohol and isopropyl alcohol are the most frequently used. They are mainly used as skin antiseptic and act by denaturing bacterial proteins, they have no action on spore or virus. They must be used in water at 60-70% concentration. Isopropyl alcohol is a better fat solvent more bactericidal and less volatile. It is used for the disinfection of clinical thermometers.

b. Formaldehyde:

It is active against the amino group in protein molecules. In aqueous solution it is markedly bactericidal and sporicidal and also has lethal affect on the virus. It is used to preserve the anatomical specimen and for destroying the anthrax spores in hair and wool. 10% formalin containing half percent sodium tetrate borats is used to sterilize clean metal instruments. Formaldehyde gas is used for sterilizing instrument and heat sensitive character. It is used for fumigating works sick room and laboratories under properly controlled condition, clothing, bedding, furniture and books can be satisfactorily disinfected.

c. Phenols:

Phenol is a powerful microicidal substance. This and other phenolic disinfectant derived from coaltar is widely used as disinfectant for various purposes in hospitals. Lysol and cresols are active agent for a wide range of organism. They are not readily inactivated by the presence of good general disinfectants. These are obtained by the distortion of coaltar between temperature of 170ºC and 270ºC. 'Lister' the father of antiseptic surgery first introduced their use in surgery. Since then a wide range of phenolic compounds as disinfectants are developed. The lethal affect of phenols is due to their capacity to cause cell membrane damage. Aqueous solution is sued in the treatment of the wounds.

d. Halogens:

Chlorine and its compound have been used as disinfectants for many years. Chlorine is most commonly used as the Hypochlorite's. Chlorine and hypochlorite are markedly bactericidal. They have a wide spectrum of activity against viruses. The organic chloramines are used as antiseptic for dressing the wounds.

C. Sterilization by physical means:

Radiation: Two types of radiations are used for sterilization purpose – non ionizing and ionizing. Infrared and ultraviolet rays are of non – ionizing energy while gamma rays are highly ionizing type.

Non-ionizing radiation:

In non-ionizing radiation electromagnetic rays, with wavelength longer, than those of visible light are used and these are to a larger extent absorbed, as heat. Hence infra red radiation can be considered as a form of air sterilization. Infra red radiation can be considered as a rapid mass of sterilization of syringes, uv radiation is used for disinfecting enclosed area such as entry ways hospital wards, operation room and small virus inoculation rooms and virus laboratories.

X-rays, Gamma rays cosmic rays are highly lethal to DNA and other vital constituents. They have a very high penetrative effect and referred as cold sterilization. High energy electron radiation as a method of sterilization is not widely used in medicine.

D. Removal of micro-organism by filtration

This is the method used to red heat level liquid of micro organism. This is useful for antibiotics solution. By this technique we can obtain bacteria free filtrates of toxin and bacteriophages. This method is also useful when we need to separate micro-organism which is scanty in fluids. The filter would retain the organisms and the filter, rise could be cultured. There are different types of filter such as:

1. Seitz filter
2. Membrane filter

1. Seitz filter: (Asbestos filter):

This method is made from the crystalline type of asbestos. Chemically this is mainly composed of magnesium silicate. The filter disc is supported by a metal mount and is inserted rough side up ensuring that the metal support grids are in position. The filter is attached to vacuum flask though a silicon rubber lung. The side arm of the flask is plugged with non absorbent cotton wool and the filter unit is wrapped in treat paper and autoclaved. After use the disc is discarded and each time a fresh disc is used. Sterilization by this method is not safe for clinical use. But this is used in the soft drink factories.

2. Membrane filter (Millipore)

Two types are gradowl membrane (grades collection membrane) is composed of cellulose nitrate and mordents are composed of cellulose acetate. The gradowl membranes are made from an acetone between of colloidal diluted with ethylalcohol. Either mixture to which are added varying amounts of Amyl alcohol. The mixture is poured into a shallow cell in a room which is in a constant temperature and allowed to evaporate from varying periods of 1-3 hrs and then washed over an extended period with distilled water. By varying the amount of composition of collection mixture and the condition of evaporation filter of average pose size (APS) ranging from 3μ to 10mμ. These filters are sterilized by autoclave at 121°C for about 15 minutes. This type of filtration is carried out in the laboratory.

Cultivation of micro-organism

It is essential to grow the organism from infected material to identify the cause of infection, only after growing them and isolating them in pure culture they can be identifies. Culture media gives artificial emulation stimulating natural condition necessary for growth.

Bacteria differ considerably in their nutritional requirement and over 7,000 cultures have been tried. The basic requirements of culture media are

    1.   Energy source
    2.   Carbon source
    3.   Nitrogen source

4. Salts such are phosphate – chlorides, carbonates of the Na, Mg, Fe and Ca and trace elements such as Mn, Mo, Cu.
5. A satisfactory pH, usually 7.2 – 7.6
6. Adequate oxidation and reduction potential.

The characteristic of an ideal culture medium age that is

1. Must give a satisfactory growth from small inoculums and orally from a single cell.
2. Should give rapid growth
3. Should be easy to prepare
4. Should be reasonably cheap and easily reproducible.
5. Should make it possible for the entire characteristic in which we are interested to be demonstrated.

Undefined ingredient used in preparation of culture media:

There are some ingredients which are commonly used in the cultivation of the microbes. The undefined ingredient includes water, Agar-agar, peptons, casein hydrolysate, meat extract, and blood serum. All these ingredients giving nutrition to the cultivating microbes as they are easily available.

Agar-agar: It is most important constituent of solid media. It is a complex polysaccharide obtained from the sea weeds. It metals at 80°C – 100°C and in acidic or alkaline pH and usually solidified at 35-42°C.

Peptone: It is complex, mixture of partially digested protein its constituents are proteases, polypeptides and variety of inorganic salt including phosphate. These peptones are usually nitrogenous material and also act as buffer.

The cultivating media is classified into two types mainly based on the chemical nature.

Based on the physical nature, the media is classified into three types: Broth, Semisolid and Solid.

i. Broth (Liquid): Bacteria grow very well in fluid media in 3-4 hours. Hence they are used as enriched media before plating on solid media. They are not suitable for the isolation of organism in pure culture. This a clear transparent straw colored fluid prepared from meat extract.

ii. Semisolid: to the above prepared liquid (both) media when 0.3% of Agar is added, the liquid solution becomes the semisolid. This media is commonly used for finding the motility of the microbes.

iii. Solid: the solid media is used to study the colonies of individual bacteria. This media is essential for the isolation of organism in pure form.

Defined / Synthetic:

These media are prepared solely from pure chemically substances and the exact composition of the system is known. These are used for various special studies such as metabolic requirement. Simple peptone, water medium, 1% peptone with 0.5% Nacl in water may be considered as semi defined medium. This media is further classified based on the composition of media like:

  i.   Simple media
  ii.   Complex media

i. Simple media: The simple media consists of peptone meat extract. Sodium chloride and water, nutrient agar, are commonly used in laboratories. If the concentration of the agar is reduced then it will become semisolid agar is obtained, which enables the motile organism to spread. Increasing the concentration of agar to 6% prevent spreading or swaring by organism such as proteins.

ii. Complex media: This media is having some added ingredient for special purpose for brooding certain special nutrients required for the growth of the bacterium. All special media come under complex media.

Artificial media:

Undefined media: this media is further subdivided into:

  a.   Enriched media
  b.   Selective media
  c.   Indicator media

a. Enriched media: In this media, substance such as blood serum, egg is added to a basal medium. This media are used to grow bacteria. This is called as enriched media (ex: blood agar, chocolate agar and egg media).

c. Selective media: If in the above media the inhabiting substance is added, to a solid medium it enables a greater number of the required bacterium to form the color. Ex desrychorate citrate medium for dysentery bacilli such solid media are known as selective media.

d. Indicator media: these media contains the indicator which changes the color when a bacterium grows in them. In cooperation of sulphate in coilson and Blair medium *S. thyphii* reduces the sulphite to sulphide in the presence of glucose. These indicators are also use to known the acidic / basic nature of the microbes.

b. Bacterial Isolation: Before isolating a pathogen the researcher has to have some basic knowledge of the pathogen and the medium in which it can grow, so that they can develop culture media and isolate the required pathogen. After an organism has attained the purposed growth in isolation medium it is usually transferred to the solid medium for colony isolation. Many methods have been derived which are as follows:

Isolation of Normal Bacteria by Plating:

i. Primary isolation by streak plate.

In situation where the microbiologist does not seek quantization the technique for isolation on solid media is usually that of stretching. This is accomplished by transferring some of the material over the surface of the solid medium in a petriplate. Most of the bacteria should separate from one another. The transfer of small portion of one of these colonies via on inoculating needle to a tube of sterile culture medium should result in growth of pure culture the streaking may be done which a needle or cotton swab or special bent glass spreader. Another procedure is to use an agar containing an indicator or substance which gives the colonies of desired organism.

ii. Isolation of variable count by spread plate:

The spread plate technique consists of pipetting the proper dilution to the surface of the solid medium plate and spreading the material evenly over the top of the plate. This is accomplished by means of a usually consists of a short small glass rod bent into an L shape to that the long arm is about 3 to 4inches in length and the short arm is about 1inch long. The dilution should be plated in triplicate in order to obtain coverage and thus least may be found.

The division of plates by a marker prior to counting my assist in counting colonies estimates the organism per ml of the original medium are then made by averaging number of colonies from plating of the proper dilution and multiplying by ten times the reciprocal of the dilution.

Powered plate with decimal dilution:

A distribution of bacteria as in the streak plate method can also be achieved by mixing the bacteria into melted agar and setting, it solidify so that the bacteria are all separated by the gilled media and form their colonies in its. This is of particular value when one wishes to enumerate the bacteria of a certain kind by counting the number of colonies, which develop from a known dilution.

PATHOGEN ENTER THE BODY VIA SKIN

Pathogen that enters the body through the skin is broadly classified into two types: pyogenic and toxigenic. Pyogenic cocci are of two types: The gram –ve and gram +ve where as the toxigenic bacteria is gram –ve. Toxogenic bacteria are again broadly classified into two types: *Bacillus anthracies* and *Clastodium* species whereas pyogenic cocci are classified into *Sciesesria, Streptococci* and *Staphelococci.*

Toxogenic Bacteria

Bacillus anthracies: (Of anthracies)

The *Bacillus anthrax* is a causative agent and is gram +ve and fast. The spores do not stain by ordinary stain. The organism will grow in complex chemically defined media. Aerobic conditions are best for growth and variation in oxygen and ratio are tolerated. But an aerobic growth can also occur.

Anthrax is a zoonosis, animals are infected by the ingrowths of the spore present in the soil. They infect on variety of animals. The disease spread from man to man is rare. The disease is generally fatal septicemia but may sometimes localized resembling the cutaneous disease in man. Infected animal shed their microbes through the mouth, nose and rectum which speculate in the soil and remain as the source of infection. Hence soil acts as reservoir substance.

Human anthrax is contracted from animal directly or indirectly. These diseases may be cutaneous, pulmonary (Respiratory) and intestinal. But all these types are leading fatal septicemia

Cutaneous: cutaneous anthrax follows entry of the bacteria through the skin, face, neck, hand arms and back as the usual site. The lesion starts as a papule, 1-3 days after infection and become vascular containing blood which may be clear or blood strained. The whole area is congested and filled which puss and arranged round a central necrotic lesion which is covered by black Escher. The lesion is called malignant pastute. The disease is common in dock workers. Cutaneous anthrax generally resolves spontaneously but may sometimes led to fatal septicemia if the patients is not treated properly the microbes enter into the lymphocytes.

Pulmonary: Pulmonary anthrax is called wool sorters disease. It is common in workers who work in wool factories due to inhalation of the dust from infected wool. This is a hemorrhagic pneumonia with a high fatality rate. Hemorrhage meningitis occurs as a complication.

Intestinal: It is rare, occurs mainly is primitive communities, who eat the cases of the animal dying of anthrax. Violent enteritis with bloody diarrhea occur with high case of fatality. These organism have a very high capacity of surviving at any type of involution therefore they form the spore. If these spores are subjected to the favorable condition they develop. Spores are commonly found in the soil and then multiple in alkaline soil and the temperature is between 15ºC to 20ºC and these organisms enters the body through small wounds.

Diagnosis: Anthrax may be diagnosed microscopically. The immunofluoresence technique can be adopted for identifying the *Bacillus anthrax*. Implement fixation and tanned cell coated antigen, agglutination technique, serological demonstration the type of test may be employed depends on the nature of the material available.

Prevention of human anthrax is mainly by general method such as improvement of factories hygiene and proper sterilization of animal products like hides and wool carcasses of animal suspected to have died of anthrax are buried tin deep in quick time, to prevent the contamination which soil. Prevention of anthrax is also aided by active immunization. The anthrax vaccine was for the first time prepared by pasture. Pasture vaccine was attenuated by growth of bacillus at 42ºC-43ºC.

Treatment: The antibiotic therapy effects in normal cases but succeed rarely. In animal as therapy is not started sufficiently early antibiotics have no effect, if ones the toxin is formed only with penicillin and streptomycin treatment case fatality in malignant pastula has been reduced from 20% to 25% scalvoi serum prepared by active immunization of assess used to be the specific treatment formerly.

CLOSTRIDIUM SPECIES

The genus *Clostridium* consist of rod shaped bacteria and these are gram +ve. Their growth is characterized in the absence of oxygen and they form the spore. The genus contains the bacteria responsible for Gas gangrene, Food poisoning and Tetanus. These three diseases are caused by the different types of *Clostridium*. *Cl. tetans* causes the tetanus and *Cl. welchii* causes the gas gangrene.

CLOSTRIDIUM TETANI

Clostridium tetani is the causative organism of tetanus. Tetanus has been known from very early time having been described by the Hepperatus scale and raltone transmitted the disease to rabbit. *Cl. Tetani* is widely distributed in soil and in the intestine of man and animals. It is cosmopolitan and has been recovered from a wide variety of other sources. These organisms utilize the glucose and release the exotoxin. This toxin affects the central nervous system, hence called as Neurotoxin. This neurotoxin has dual affect. It affects on the peripheral motor nerves and the spinal cord (increase reflex inhibiting).

The most characteristic reaction to the toxin in muscle contraction is s own down as a result the muscle of jaw locked. Hence the disease is also called as the "locked jaw" swallowing of the muscle of the neck by a slight sound the patient fearing opisthotnous condition is seen.

Diagnosis: Laboratory diagnosis maybe made by demonstration by microscopic culture. Isolation is more likely from excide buts of tissue from the enrobe depth of would than from wound swards or diagnosis is also may be the animal inoculation.

Prevention: The disease is due to the action of the toxin knee the obvious and most dependable method of prevention is to build up antitoxic immunity by active immunization. The nature of the treatment mainly depends on the type of wound the immune status to the patient. The available method of propyylaxmi (treatment) is surgical attention. The prevention of this disease includes vaccine such as anti serum (ATS).

Treatment: The patient should be treated in hospital preferably in special unit. The reason for this is to protect them from noise and light which may provoke convulsions.

Clostridum Welchii:

It is normal inhabitant of the large intestine of man and animals. It is found is faces and contaminates within the skin of the perincum and bullocks and though the spore are commonly found in dust, air and soil.

It is a gram +ve with straight parallel side and rounded or hemicaled ends about 4 – 6.4 x 24. It is polymorphic and filamentous and involution forms are common. It is capsulated and non-motile; spores are central or subterminal but are rarely seen in a artificial culture or in material from pathogenically lesion.

Clostradium welchii causes many diseases, but the most common is gas gangrene. This disease is more common in military person. This disease is caused by the injury or nail prick or bullet prick. If this injury is deeper than only the microbes multiply very fast therefore their condition is anaerobic, more suitable for multiplication and leads to formation of puss.

Diagnosis: The diagnosis of gas gangrene must be made primarily in clinical ground and the function of the laboratory is only to provide confirmation of the clinical diagnosis. Bacteriological examination also helps to differentiate gas gangrene. The species to be collected are

1. The films from the muscles at the edges of the affected area from the tissue in the vecrotic area from the exudates in the deeper parts of the wound.
2. Exudates from the parts where the infection appears. For this the most important test is the stormy fermentation test.

Treatment: Surgery is the most prophylactic and therapeutic measures in the gas gangrene. All the damaged tissue should be removed promptly and the wound irrigated to remove blood, necrotic tissue and foreign material. Chemotherapy and antibiotic are of value in prophylaxes in combination with adequate surgery. Gas gangrene is susceptible to sulphnamide metronidiaide pencillus and tetracycline. Antibacterial therapy appeared to be of little benefit in the treatment of the established gas gangrene.

Prevention: Sterile immunization with toxoids has been found experimentally to induce good antitoxin response, but the utility of this method in prophylaxis is uncertain

UNIT – III

Unit – III

Entamoeba histolytica

Phylum:	Sarcomastigophora
Subphylum:	Sarcodina
Class:	Lobosea
Order:	Amoebida
Family:	Endamoebidae
Genus:	*Entamoeba*
Species:	*histolytica*

I. Introduction:

Certainly closely related forms of Amoeba, known under different generic names are found to lead a parasitic mode of life in the intestine of man and other animals. The human beings may be infected by the species of Entamoeba, Endolimax, Iodamoeba and Dientomoeba of these *Entamoeba histolytica* (Entos = within; amoeba = change; histos = tissue; lysis = dissolve) is the pathogenic responsible for the disease Amoebiasis or amoebic dysentery in man. The other species of *Entamoeba* like *E.coli* and *E.gingivalis* are described to be non-pathogenic.

II. Geographical distribution:

World-wide, more common in the tropics and sub-tropics than in the temperate zone. The more epidemic conditions of this parasite are reported from Mexico, China. India, Philippines, South Africa and Thailand. Its incidence is relatively higher in rural and densely populated urban areas particularly in those areas where the sanitary conditions are poor. The children and adults are more frequently infected surprisingly; the males are more commonly infected than females.

III. Habitat:

Trophozoites and *E. histolytica* (the "large race" or the tissue invading forms) live in the mucous and submucous layers of the large intestine of man.

IV. Morphology:

The structural characters of the parasite can be studied both in unstained and stained preparations (iodine and iron haematoxyline). The morphology of the three phases in the life cycle of *E. histolytica* is described.

(i) Trophozoite (The growing the feeding stage): Under the microscope, the living parasite, in a warm stage, is seen to exhibit slow gliding movement. The clear hyaline ectoplasm had a jerky movement. The clear hyaline ectoplasm has a jerky movement, flowing in the whole granular endoplasm. The morphological characteristics are as follows:

Shape is not fixed because of constantly changing position. Size ranges from 18 to 40µm average being 20 o 30µm. The cytoplasm is divisible into two portions a clear ectoplasm and a granular endoplasm. Red blood cells, leucocytes and tissue debris are found inside the endoplasm. Nucleus is spherical in shape and varying in size from 4 to 6µm. Nucleus occupies an eccentric position inside the body of the parasite. In stained preparations the nuclear structure shows karyosome, nuclear membrane, nucleoplsmic striations etc.

ii. Pre-cystic stage: It is smaller in size. Varying from 10 to 20 μm. It is round or slightly avoid with a blunt pseudopodium projecting from the periphery. The endoplasm is free of red blood cells and other ingested food particles; larger nuclear structure retains the characteristics of the trophozoite.

iii. Cystic stage: A mature cyst is a quadrinucleate spherical body, its cytoplasm is clear and hyaline, and the nuclear structure retaining the characters of the trophozoite. The cyst varies greatly in size – the "small race" being 6 to 9 μm and the large race 12 to 15 μm.

The cyst begins as a uninucleate body but soon divides by primary fission and develops into binucleate and quadrinucleate bodies. The single nucleus multiple and forms quadrinucleate. The nuclei undergo gradual reduction in size, becoming 2μm in diameters during the process of division. The cytoplasm of the cyst shows in early stage of development, the following chromotoid or chromidial bars and glycogen mass. Immature cysts passed in the faces may however complete their development outside.

Methods of Reproduction: Excystation, Encystation and Multiplication

Excystation: This is the process of transformation of cysts to trophozoites and occurs only when the cysts enter into the alimentary canal of man.

Encystation: This is the process of transformation of trophozoites to cyst and occurs in the lumen of the intestine of an infected individual.

Multiplication: This occurs only in the trophozoite phase. Reproduction of trophozoites occurs by simple binary fission.

V. Cultivation

A successful culture of *E. histolytica* was first made by Beeck and Drbohlow (1925) using solidified blood agar or solidified egg slopes covered with Locke's solution. The growth of *E. histolytica* requires in culture the presence of starch or rice flour and some metabolic associates, such as enteric bacteria, organism or the parasitic flagellate *T. cruzi*, living or dead.

VI. Immunology

Certain serological test, such as complement fixation test, precipitation test, immobilization test of *E. histolytica* with hyper-immune sera of rabbits and reaction of *E. histolytica* with fluarescin – tagged homologous antibody suggests the development of specific immune bodies in the sera of individual who has recovered from amoebiasis, particularly invasive (hepatic) amoebiasis. Such humoral antibodies however do not protect the individual who has recovered from amoebiasis against re-infection.

VII. Life Cycle:

E. histolytica passes its life cycle only in on host, the man. There are mainly two phases of development trophozoite and cyst with a transitory stage of pre-cystic form.

The mature quadrinucleated cysts are the infective forms of the parasite. When these cysts are swallowed along with the contaminated food and drink by a susceptible person. They are capable of further development inside the gut. The fully developed cysts thus gain the entrance into the alimentary canal, pass unaltered through the stomach. The cyst wall is resistant to the action of gastric juice but is digested by the action of trypsin in the intestine. The excystation occurs when the cyst reaches the caecum or the lower part of the ileum. Each cyst liberate a single amoeba with four nuclei, a tetranucleate amoeba which forms and amoebulae (metacycstic trophozoites). The young amoebulae, invade the tissues and ultimately lodge in the submucous tissue of the large gut, their normal habitat. Here they grow and multiply by binary fission. It is to be noted that trophozoite phase is responsible for producing lesions of amoebiasis.

During growth, *E. histolytica* a proteolytic ferment of the nature of histolysin which brings about destruction and necrosis of tissues and thereby helps the parasite in obtaining nourishment. *E. histolytica* wonder about in the tissues of the gut wall entering into the deeper layers and sometimes find their way into the portal vein to be carried away to the liver. In liver the trophic forms may for a time grow and multiply but encystations does not occur, because so far as its biological aspect is concerned it has reached a dead end.

There parasites which remain in the intestinal wall may cause an attack of acute dysentery, in which a large numbers of trophozoites are discharged along with the slough. This again is also to the species itself because they are causing acute dysentery it may completely exterminate its own race. A high degree of Pathogenicity of the parasite is obviously a disadvantage to itself.

After sometimes, increase in the tolerance of the host, the lesions become quiescent and commence to heal. The parasite now finds it difficult to continue its life cycle rarely in the trophozoite stage; so some of these trophozoites are discharged into the lumen of the bowel and are transformed into small pre-cystic forms from which the cysts are developed.

The mature quadrinucleate cysts are the most resistant and infective forms of the parasite and are particularly developed when a state of equilibrium has been established between the host and the parasite. But the cysts produced in an infected individual are unable to develop in the host in which they are produced and therefore necessitate transference to another host, where they can grow of continue their life cycle.

VIII. Reservoirs of infection and modes of infection:

Natural infection of *E. histolytica* is seen only among men and monkeys. Hence man is the commonest course of infection.

Modes infection: transmission of *E. histolytica* from man to man is effected through its encysted state and infection occurs through the ingestion of these cysts. Mature quadrinucleate cysts are the infective forms of this parasite. Fecal contamination of drinking water, vegetables and food are the primary causes. Eating of uncooked vegetables and fruits which have been fertilized with infected human faces has often led to occurrence of the disease. Occasionally drinking water supply contaminated with infected faeces gives rise to epidermis.

Role of Carriers: Handling of food by infected individuals (Cyst passes or cyst carriers) appears to be a very common method. There are two types of carriers - "contact" and "Covalecent". The former are so-called "healthy" carriers who have never suffered from amoebic dysentery. The latter are those who have recovered from a clinical attack of acute amoebic dysentery.

House-files and cockroaches which also serve as a source of infection.

IX Pathogenicity:

E. histolytica causes amoebic dysentery, abscesses in liver, lungs and brain and non-dysenteric infection. Incubation period is generally 4 to 5 days.

i) Amoebic dysentery: *E. histolytica* secretes a tissue dissolving enzyme that destroys the epithelial lining of the colon and causes its necrosis and forms the abscesses (small wounds) which later become bleeding ulcers. The ulcers vary greatly in number and size, which may produce serve dysentery. In amoebic dysentery the stools is acidic and contains pure blood and mucus, in which swarms of amoeba and blood corpuscles, are usually present. The patient feels discomfort due to the rectal straining and intense gripping pains with the passage of blood and mucus stools every few minutes.

ii) Abscesses in liver, lungs and brain: Sometimes *E. histolytica* may be drawn into the portal circulation and carried to the liver. In liver the parasite settle, attack the liver tissue and form abscesses. The patient has pain in liver region, fever and high leucocytes number, a condition referred to as amoebic hepatitis. Lung abscesses are fairly frequent; those are usually caused by direct extension from a liver abscess through the diaphragm. The lung abscesses usually rupture into a bronchial tube and discharge a brown mucous material which is coughed out with the spectrum. Sometimes the parasite also forms abscesses in the brain. Abscesses elsewhere are rare.

iii) Non-dysenteric infections: Although amoebiasis is usually thought of dysentery with blood and mucus containing stools. These conditions are exception rather than rule, many workers reported that 90% of dysentery in temperate climates are symptomless. Even in tropics dysentery is exceptional.

Population infected with *E. histolytica*, yet most of when are carriers (or) passes. The symptoms commonly associated with chronic amoebiasis are abdominal pain, nausea, and bowel irregularity, with headaches, fatigability and nervousness in minority of cases.

Symptoms: The infection of *E. histolytica* causes amoebiasis; the common symptoms are the passing out of stool with blood and mucus, abdominal pain, nausea, flatulence and bowel irregularity with headache and fatigability etc.

X. Diagnosis:

The microscopic examination of the stool of an infected man shows the presence of trophozoites and cysts in it. The presence of stone- shaped, white colored crystals of charcot-Leyden suggests the infection of *E. histolytica*. The red blood cells are clumped and are reddish-yellow or yellowish –green in color.

Microscopic or naked eye appearance: An offensive dark brown semi fluid stool. Acid in reaction, mixed with blood, mucus and much faecal matter is representative of a case of amoebic dysentery.

XI. Treatment

For prompt relief of acute or subacute dysentery the injections of Emctin are given. But certain antibiotics. Such as Fumagillin, Terramycin, Erythromycin and Aureomycin are more effective and may be given orally. For eradication of intestinal infections or in chronic cases certain arsenic compounds and a number of iodine compounds are effective. For amoebiasis of liver or lungs choroquine is quite effective. The most significant advancement in the treatment of amoebiasis is the use of Metronidazole and Tinidazole as both luminal and tissue amoebicide.

XII. Prophylaxis:

For personal prophylaxis

    i.   Use of boiled drinking water
    ii.   Protection of all food and drink from contamination by files, cockroaches and rats.
    iii.   Avoidance of use of vegetables and fruits
    iv.   Personal cleanliness and elementary hygiene conditions are to be observed while taking meals.

For community Prophylaxis

    i.   Effective sanitary disposal of faces.
    ii.   Protection of water supplies from faecal pollution
    iii.   Avoidance of the use of human excrement as fertilizer
    iv.   Detection and isolation of carriers.

II. Giardiasis

Phylum: Sarcomastigophora
Subphylum: Mastigophora
Class: Zoomastigophora
Order: Diplomonadida
Family: Hexamitidae
Genus: *Giardia*
Species: *lamblia*

I. Introduction:

Giardia lamblia was first seen by Leeuwenhoek (1681) while examining stool. It is also called *G. lambila* (Old name Lambila) is a parasite in the small intestine and colon of man.

II. Geographical distribution: World – Wide

III. Habitat: Duodenum and the upper part of the jejunum of man.

IV. Morphology: Exists in the phases – trophozoite and cyst.

Trophozoites: When viewed flat the shape of the trophozoite is like that of a tennis or badminton racket and when viewed side-on it resembles a longitudinally split pear. The dorsal surface it convex and the ventral surface is concave with a sucking disc. The life of the trophozoite is 14 µm long by 7µm broad. The anterior end is broad and rounded and the posterior end tapers to a sharp point. It is bilaterally symmetrical and all organs of the body are paired. Thus there are three axostyles, two nuclei and four pairs of flagella.

Cyst: The fully formed cyst is oval in shape and measures 12μm long by 7μm broad. The axostyles lie more or less diagonally forming a last of dividing line within the cyst – wall. There are four nuclei which may remain clustered at one end or lie in pairs at opposite poles. The remains of the flagella and the margins of the sucking disk may be seen inside the cytoplasm. An acid environment often causes the parasite to encyst.

V. Cultivation

It grows well on medium of chick embryo extract, human serum. Hettinger's digest (Trypitc must digest) and Hank's solution.

VI. Life cycle:

In the trophozoite stage are parasite multiples in the intestine of man by binary fission when conditions in the duodenum are unfavorable, encystment occurs, usually in the large intestine. During encystment a thick resistant wall is recreated by the parasites and the cell them divides into two within the cyst. Infection of man is brought about the ingestion of cysts. Within 30 minutes of ingestion, the cyst hatches out two trophozoites, which then multiply in enormous number and colonies in the duodenum. To avoid the high activity of duodenum *Giardia* often localizes in the biliary tract (Gall bladder).

VII. Pathogenicity:

With the help of sucking disc the parasite attaches itself on to this convex surface of the epithelial cells in the intestine and may cause a disturbance of intestinal function, leading to malabsorption of fat. Consequently the patient may complain of persistent looseness of bowels and mild steatorrhoea (Passage of yellowish and gray stools in which there is excess of fat). The parasite is also capable of producing harm by its toxic effect (allergy), traumatic and irritative effect as well as by spoliative action, i.e., by diverting nutrients, clinically the cases may be divided as follows:

1. Silent cases without any symptoms
2. Intestinal: Chronic enteritis and acute – entero – colitis
3.   General: Fever, anemia and allergic manifestations
4. Chronic cholecystopathy

VIII. Diagnosis:

a. Microscopical examinations of a freshly passed stool fix the demonstration of *Giardia* trophozoites and cyst; the former are found in a diarrheic stool or after a purgative.
b. *Giardia* trophozoites may be recovered both in the bile A (aspirated from duodenum) and B drawn by duodenal incubation.

IX. Treatment:

Alberin and acranil have been found to be the specific for Giardiasis. Schneider (161) reported good results with a derivative of indiazole (metronidazole). Chloroquine in doses of 300 mg base once daily for 5 days is also effective.

III. Trypanosominasis of man and domestic animals:

Phylum:	Sarcomastigophora
Subphylum:	Mastigophora
Class:	Zoomastigophora
Order:	Kinetplastida
Family:	Trypanosomatidae
Genus:	*Trypanosoma*
Species:	*gambiense*

I. Introduction:

The genus trypanosoma is a parasitic in the blood of many vertebrates like fishes, amphibians, reptiles, birds and mammals. The disease caused by trypanosoma is called Trypanosominasis. *Trypanosoma gambiense* and *T. rhodesience* live as parasite in the human blood and cause a deadly disease known as sleeping sickness in Africa.

II. Geographical distribution:

The different species of trypanosoma are reported from central and West Africa, Congo and Central America, Commonly areas near the rivers and lakes having low marshy land have the greatest incidence of infection because the insect vector inhabits in these areas.

III. Habitat:

Trypanosoma gambiense lives as parasite is the blood, lymph, lymph nodes, spleen or cerebrospinal fluid of man and in the intestine of blood – sucking fly *Glossina palpalis* (Tse tse fly).

IV. Morphology:

T. gambiense exists in the vertebrate hosts as a trypomastigote from. It is an elongated rather than flattened spindle shaped. Its colorless, sickle shaped and flattened microscopic body. The anterior end is more pointed and the posterior end is blunt. It s body length varies from 15 to 30µ and width from 1 to 3µ. The flagellum starts from the posterior extremity near the kintoplast, curves around the body in the form of an undulating membrane and continues as a free flagellum. It is an actively motile flagellate.

Polymorphism: Trypanosoma is a polymorphic form. Hoare has notice six morphological stages. These forms have been named mostly on the basis of the arrangement of flagellum viz. amastigote (Lushamarial), promastigote (Leptomonad), promastogote (Leptomonad) Epimastigatoe (Critihidial) and trypomastigote (Trypanosome). Of the four forms three are having flagellum and one not having flagellums.

V. Staining reaction:

When stained with Remanowsky stain, the cytoplasm and the undulating membrane appear pale blue, the nucleus reddish purple or red; the kinetoplast and the flagellum dark red.

VI. Cultivation:

It has been cultivated in a medium of Ringer's solution with sodium chloride, Tyrode's solution and citrated human blood, long slender forms of trypomastigote. Similar to mid-gut forms of testse fly are encountered in culture.

VII. Immunology:

T. Gambiense infection both in animals and man stimulates the output of large quantities of immunoglobulin; most of it is in non-specific IgM rather than in the IgG, having no affinity for the infecting organism. The host is unable to produce specific protective antibody to "large" antigens or the antibody producing cells do not receive any message from macrophages to go into action.

It is also known that the African trypanosome is associated with profound immune-suppressive effects. The humoral immune response is so reversely depressed that the patient will not be able to resist any bacterial invasion.

VIII. Life-cycle:

T. gambiense passes its life-cycle in two different hosts. The vertebrate hosts (definitive host) are man and domestic animals. The insect (Intermediate host) are several species of the tests fly (Glossina).

Development in man and other vertebrate hosts:

The metacycstic stage (infective form) of trypomastigote are introduced by the bite of infected *Glossina* develop into long, slender forms and multiple by binary longitudinal fission at one site of inoculation. These become stumpy via "Intermediate" forms. Subsequently the parasites invade the blood streams, resulting in parasitanemia. The trypomastigote forms are taken up by the tsetse fly along with its blood-meal and undergo a series of complex biological development inside the insect host before becoming infective to man.

Development in tsetse fly: The short stumpy forms of trypomastigate ingested by the insect, first change their morphology in the mid-gut long slender forms (the kinetoplast lying mid-way between the nucleus and the posterior end) appear which pass to the posterior end of the extra – peritrophic space (a space between the peritrophic membrane and the epithelial cells), where they continue to multiple for some days. By the 15th day they escape from the anterior end of this space and enter the lumen of the proventriculus (the proventricular form is same as that of the mid-gut form). Then they migrate forwards to the buccal cavity, pass on to the hypoharynx and eventually reach the salivary gland through the opening of the salivary ducts. Here they multiply and change their morphology, first into epimastigote and then into metacyclic stage (short stumpy forms of trypomastigote) which are infective to man.

The time taken for the complete evolution of the infective forms (metacyclic forms) inside the tsetse fly is about 20 days. These tsetse flies remain infective for the rest of their lives, a period extending up to 185 days. There is no evidence of a hereditary transmission of trypanosome in the fly to its offspring.

IX. Transmitting agents and Reservoirs of Infection:

The animal strains of T. Gambiense is transmitted by Glossina moritans amongst domestic animals. Glossima palpali is the transmitting agents amongst man. G. palpalis feeds on blood of man. There are shade and moisture loving flies and found in scrubs and shady trees near water (there are called reverie species). They do not travel far from their breeding grounds. Animals receviors of infection for this strain are not yet definitely known. Domestic pigs "gambience" strain is concerned man himself is the reservoir of infection. Interchange of trypanosomes between tretse fly and man takes place w near the water – supply of the village.

X. Pathogenesis:

The bite of an infected fly is usually followed by itching and irritation near the wound, and frequently a local dark red lesion develops. In blood the parasite multiples and absorbs nutrients from it. After a few days, fever and headache develops, recurring at regular intervals accompanied by increasing weakness, loss of weight and anemia. Usually the parasite succeeds in penetrating the lymphatic glands. Because of its infection the lymphatic glands swell and after it the parasites enter the cerebrospinal fluid and brain causing a sleeping sickness like condition. Development of lethargic condition and recurrence of fever are the symptoms of its infection.

XI. Disease:

Trypanosoma causes Trypanosominasis; most commonly referred to sleeping sickness leading to coma stage and finally resulting into the death of the patient. In fact, two types of diseases are formed by Trypanosome which are essentially similar is symptoms. There are Gambian and Rhodesian sleeping sickness. The only difference between two is that the later is more rapid causing the death of the patients within 3-4 months of infection.

XII. Diagnosis:

The diagnosis is confirmed by examining fresh or stained peripheral blood or by examining the cerebrospinal fluid obtained by lumbar puncture or by examining the extract of enlarged lymphatic glands.

XIII. Treatment:

Arsenic and antimony compounds were until recently the drugs for treatment of Trypanosominasis, but now they are rarely used except for late stages when the parasite has invaded the central nervous system. The drugs Bayer 205 (also called Antrypol; Germanin or Suramin) and pentamidine or lomidine are new widely used for both treatment and now widely used for both treatment and prophylaxis of human infections. These drugs are low in toxicity, effective in treatment, and prevent reinfection for several months.

XIV. Prophylaxis:

The following measures are suggested for preventing the infection of this parasite.

1. By eradicating the vectors: The infection of this parasite can be checked by completely eradicating the secondary host (Tsetse fly). For this, endemic areas should be kept clean and regular spray of insecticides like DDT is suggested which helps in eradicating the fly.
2. Care should be taken to keep the reservoir host free from its infection.
3. Prevention medicines should be taken frequently and periodically which helps to a great extent from its infection.

Haemosporidians of man and domestic animals

Classification

Phylum: Apicomplexa

Class: Aconoidasida

Order: Haemosporida

Family: Plasmodiidae

Genus: *Plasmodium*

Species: *vivax*

I. Generic characters:

The parasites belonging to this genus possess a life cycle which shows an alternation of generation accompanied by an alteration of host. Asexual cycle (cycle of schizogony) occurs inside the red blood cells of the vertebrate most and sexual cycle (Cycle of sporogony) occurs in an invertebrate host. The product of schizogony is called a merozoite and the product of sporogomy is called a sporozoite. The gametogony (formation of gametocytes) really starts inside the red blood cells of the vertebrate host and is completed in various species of blood sucking mosquitoes with the production of sporozoite the forms infective to the vertebrate host.

Parasites of man

Four recognized and district species are:

    i.   *Plasmodium malariae*

    ii. *Plasmodium vivax*

    iii.   *Plasmodium falciparum*
    iv.   *Plasmodium ovale*

II. Malaria parasite of man:

Geographical distribution: Malaria parasites are found in all countries, extending from 40°s to 60°N. The tropical zone *P. malariae* is parasite of sub-tropical zone. *P. vivax* is the prevailing species of the temperate zone. The distribution of *P. Ovale* has mainly been reported from East Africa, West Africa especially Nigeria and Philippines.

Habitat: The malarial parasites infecting man, after passing through a developmental phase in the parenchyma cells of the liver, reside inside the red blood corpuscles and are carried by the circulating blood to all the organs.

III. Human cycle:

Human cycle starts with the introduction of sporozoite by the bite of an infected female anopheles mosquito. It comprises the following stages:

i. Pre-erythrocytic Schizogony:

Sporozoite does not directly enter into a red blood corpuscle to start its erythrocytic schizogony but undergoes development inside the tissues of man. This phase is called pre-erythrocytic schizont; the cycle lasts for 8 days in *P. vivax*, 6 days in *P. falciparum* and 9 days in *P. Ovale*. The pre-erythrocytic Schizogony occurs inside the parenchyma cells of the liver. The liberated merozoites are called cryptozoties.

The smaller ones (merozoites) enter the circulation and the larger ones (macromesozoites) re-enter the liver cells.

ii. Erythrocytic Schizogony: During this phase the parasites resides inside the red blood corpuscle and passes through the stages of trophozoite, schizont and merozoite. The parasitic multiplication during the erythrocytic phase is responsible for bringing on a clinical attack of malaria. The cycle starts for 48 hours.

iii. Gametogony: Some of the merozoites instead of developing into trophozoites and schizonts give rise to forms which are capable of sexual function after leaving the human host. There are called gametocytes. Only the mature gametocytes are found in the peripheral blood. The maturation is completed in about 96 hours (4 days). Gametocytes do not cause any febrile reaction in the human host. The individual who harbors the gametocytes is known as "Carrier".

iv. Exo-Erythrocytic Schizogony: After establishment of blood infection the initial pre-erythrocytic phase disappears completely in *P. falciparum*, whereas it persistence in the form of local immunity in other species. The persistence of this phase is exo-erythrocytic schizogony and is now held to be responsible for relapses of vivax, ovale and quartan malaria. The merozoites liberated from the exo-erythrocytic schizogony are collectively called phanerozoites.

The following scheme represents the tissue phase of *P. vivax, P. malariae* and *P.ovale*.

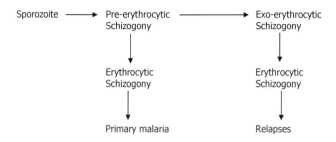

The following scheme represents the tissue phase of *P. falciparum*:

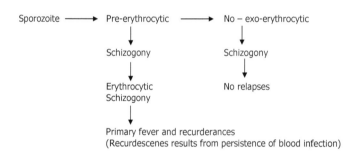

IV. Mosquito Cycle: (Sexual cycle of parasite)

The sexual cycle of malarial parasite first starts in the human host by the formation of gametocyte. When a female Anopheles sucks the blood meal of an infected person it ingests both the sexual and asexual forms; but the sexual form develops where as the asexual forms die of immediately. The carrier must contain at least 12 gametocytes per mm^3 of blood and the number of female gametocytes must be in excess.

The first phase of development occurs inside the mid-gut (Stomach) of the mosquito. The maturation occurring by a process of nuclear reduction and extrusion of polar bodies. The gametes are ready for fertilization and by a process of chemo taxis the microgamete are attracted towards macrogamete. One of the male gamete attaches to the periphery of the female gametes the resulting body is called zygote.

In the next 24 hours, the zygote lengthens and matures into an ookinete (formerly called a vermicule). The entry of the ookinete into the cell is made possible by the recreation of proteolytic substance which causes lysis of the cell membrane; where it develops into an oocyte.

The oocyte is a spherical mass surrounded by structure capsules; it measures 12 cm in diameter. As the oocyste matures, meiotic and mitotic division follow to form large number of sporozoite. Oocyte ruptures, releasing sporozoite in the body cavity of the mosquito. They have a special predilection towards the salivary glands ultimately reach in maximum number into the ducts. The mosquito at this stage is capable of transmitting infection through mass sporozoite in the salivary glands is to be taken as proof of the development of the human malarial parasite.

V. Reservoirs of Infection

Human species of malarial parasites are not harbored by any of the lower animals. Hence man, particularly the children in an endemic area, acts as the only reservoir of infection. In some part of Africa chimpanzees may act as reservoir for the malaria.

VI. Method of transmission and spread of malaria:

The of Anopheles mosquitoes acts a intermediate in transmitting infection to man. The malaria parasite undergoes developmental changes in the mosquito. The infection is transmitted by the inoculation method. During the act of biting, the mosquito's proboscis pierces the skin and the salivary secretion is injected into the punctured wound which is directly introduced into the blood stream but cannot be found in it after about half an hour.

Spread of Malaria:

The factors responsible for the spread of malaria include:

1. The presence of a gametocyte (cover source of malaria parasite)
2. Existence of a suitable Anopheles vector and
3. Susceptible person

VII. Pathogenicity:

Infection with the *Plasmodium* causes intermitted fevers which are known as malaria. Each of the four species causes a characteristics fever and the diseases are

P. vivax – *vivax* malaria (Benign tentain malaria)
P. malariae – quartan malaria (Malariae malaria)
P. falciparum – *Falciparum* malaria
(Malignant testitain malaria)
P. ovale – *ovale* malaria

VIII. Incubation period:

The sporozoite after gaining entrance into the human body undergoes a developmental cycle first in liver and than in the RBC; brings about the onset of fever. This period of development is called the incubation period which varies with different species as follows.

P.vivax, P.ovale and P. falciparum – 10-14 days
P. malariae it is 18 days to 6 weeks

Clinical features of malaria

The main clinical manifestations in a typical case are a series of febrils paroxysms, followed by anemia and spleen enlargement.

Febrils paroxysms: the malarial paroxysm starts generally in the early afternoon but actually it may starts at any time. Each paroxysm shows a succession of 3 stages.

i.   The cold stage (lasting 20 minutes to an hour)
ii. The hot stage (lasting 1 to 4 hrs)
iii. The sweating stage (lasting 2 to 3 hours)

Thus the total duration of the febrile cycle is from 6 to 10 hrs varying however with the species of plasmodia.

Types of fever: The febrile paroxysm supchronized with the erythrocytic schizogony of the malaria parasite.

a. with a 48 hrs cycle, the fever reoccurs every third day – tertian fever

b. with a 72 hours cycle, the fever reoccurs every fourth day – quartan fever

c. Fever reoccurring at intervals of 24 hours, quotidian periodicity has also been observed.

Anemia: After a few paroxysms, anemia of a microcystic or a normocytic hypo chronic type develops as a result of breaking down of RBC's during segmentation of parasites.

Splenomegaly: Enlargement of the spleen is one of the physical signs in malaria. In primary cases the enlargement is so slight as to escape detection by palpation. After some paroxysms and usually by the second week, it is definitely enlarged and palpable.

IX. Malarial pathology:

i. Pigmentation of various organs, giving the characteristics state grey or black color. The pigment granules are physiologically inert and take no pat is the pathogenesis of malaria.

ii. Hyperplasia of the reticule – endothelial system (proliferation of cells and reticulum fibrils)

iii. Parasitized erythrocytes fitting the luminal of the capillaries of the internal organs.

iv. Degenerative changes of parenchyma cells, resulting capillary blockage

v. Immune suppression has been noticed in malarial infection.

X. Pathological changes in various organs:

Spleen: The spleen functions in malaria as a filter for removing the parasites and their product of Schizogony from the blood stream.

i.   The organ moderately enlarged
ii.   The color is state grey or black, depending on the among of pigment
iii.   The capsule is thin and stretched
iv.   Macrophage cells are greatly increased
v.   Malphigian corpuscles are free from pigments and parasites

Liver: the organ is uniformly enlarged

i.   The color varies from dark chocolate red to state grey
ii.   The cut surface shows dilated lobular reins
iii.   The kupffer cells are increased in number and cytoplasm filled with malarial pigment.

Bone marrow

i.   In acute cases the marrow of the long bones undergoes very little change.
ii.   In chronic areas the upper and lower thirds of the long bones are reddish brown in color or even state – grey or block.
iii.   Hyperplasia of R.E. cells.

Kidneys:

i. An attack of acute falciparum malaria and also in black water fever is the renal anoxia syndrome.

XI. Laboratory diagnosis of malaria:

A microscopical examination of blood film forms one of the most important diagnostic procedures in malaria. It is a good practice to take both thin and thick films; at the sametime either on the same slide or on two different slides, then the thick film and thin film examined for identifying species. In a well stained film, if parasites are numerous, the species can be easily identified.

XII. Treatment:

The various antimalarial drugs are grouped as:

1. Essential therapeutic (clinical are): 4 – ameroquinalines such as choroquine and amodiaguine, quinine and mepacrine are used for radical can 8- amino-quidnoline, primaguine is useful after the clinical cure.
2. Protective or prophylactic: Pyrimethamine and thimethprine choroquine, a metabolite of proguanil may be used as a long-acting injectable prophylactic.
3. Synergists: Sulphnamide and sulphones are often used in combination with dihdyrofolate reductase inhibitors.

XIII. Prophylaxis:

For personal prophylaxis

    i.   Protection against mosquito bites and

    ii.   Systemic use of antimalarial drugs as a prophylactic measure

For community Prophylaxis:

    i.   Prevention of carrier by antimalarial drugs

    ii.   Anti-mosquito measures

        a.   Destruction of adult mosquitoes by spraying with insecticides such as D.D.T.

        b.   Anti-larval measures consist of elimination of breading places.

UNIT – IV

PATHOGENIC NEMATODES

Trichinella spiralis

Phylum:	Nematoda
Class:	Adenophorea
Order:	Trichocephalida
Superfamily:	Trichinelloidea
Genus:	*Trichinella*
Species:	*spiralis*

I. Introduction (Common name: Trichina worm):

Trichinella spiralis or the trichinae worm is the causative agent of trichinosis; was first observed in 1821 in the muscle of patient at autopsy. Owen in 1835 described the encysted larval from in muscles of named it Trichina spiralis. The name Trichinella is derived from the mixture size of the adult, from thick hair and -ella suffix for diminutive; spiralis refers to the spirally coiled appearance of larvae in muscle.

II. Geographical distribution

Trichinosis is recognized as a important public health problem is Europe and America, but is much less common is the tropics. In Asia, the disease has been reported from Malaysia, Vietnam, Thailand china and Syria. Human trichinosis has not been recorded in India, though the larvae have been reported in animals on a few occasions.

III. Habitat:

It starts as an intestinal parasite, remaining buried in the duodenal or jejuna mucosa, where its adult life is passed but its stay there is relatively short. The fertilized female discharges embryos into the circulating blood which ultimately encyst in the striated muscles of the animal harboring the adult worm, such as the pig, rat or man.

IV. Morphology:

  a. Adult worm: It is one of the smallest nematodes infecting man. Male measures 1.4 to 1.6 mm in length with diameter of 0.04 mm. The spiecule and the copulatory sheath are lacking but at the tail end there are two conspicuous conical papillae on either side. The female is much longer than the male, measuring 3 to 4 mm in length by 0.06mm in breath. The females are viviparous and discharge embryos instead of eggs.

  b. Larvae: These measures 100μm by 6 μm. They remain encysted in the striated muscle (not cardiac or smooth muscle) of the host. Inside the cyst, the larva continues to develop up to the stage of sexual differentiation and when fully grown, it becomes ten times its original size i.e. from 100μm to 1000μm in length. The maximum size is attained by the 35th day (One larvae in a single cyst).

  c. Life span: Life span of the adult worm is very short. The male dies after fertilizing the disease about one week after infection. The female also dies after about 16 weeks, the period required for discharging larvae. The majority of the larvae encysted is muscles dies within 6 months but some may live for many years (10 to 31 years).

V. Life Cycle:

The life cycle is initiated when encysted muscle larvae are ingested. These are liberated within a few hours by the digestive processes and the first two moults are completed within 26 hours and the fourth moult in less than two days in the small intestine of the host. Development of adult stage is rapid, being completed in four days. Copulation occurs about 40 hours after infection. After copulation has taken place in the intestine the female dies and male penetrates into the mucous via liberkihns glands and some may reach the lymph spaces. Here they produce, over a period of several weeks, eggs than hatch inside the uterus of the worm.

In experimental infections a marked loss of adults occurs about the 12th day of infection; however, this depends on the animals and adults may live as long as 16 weeks in man. Some larvae may be passed in the faces during this stage of adult infection.

The first larvae (newborn larvae), which are about 0.1 mm long enter the lymph and pass in it by way of the thoracic duct to the left superior vena cava and thus reach the blood, by which they are distributed all over the body. They develop further, especially in the voluntary muscle, especially those of the diaphragm, tongue, larynx, eye and the masticator and intercostals muscles. They have also been found in the liver, pancreas and kidney.

The larvae enter striated muscle fibers and become surrounded by a capsule formed from the muscle fiber. Following penetration of the muscle cell is a modulation or dedifferentiation in the structure of the muscle cell. It is lumped a nurse cell and probably serves in larval nutrition and in the handling of nuclei and an increase in nuclear material; there is an increase in the number no of mitochondria but these are smaller than those seen in the normal muscle fiber. The myofilaments disappear and these is a marked proliferation of the sareoplasmic reticulum, particularly RER; by 10 days of infection the outer plasma membrane is highly hypervoluted and shows a 36-fold increase in the volume of the glycocalyse while a host derived double membrane completely surrounds the larva. The larvae grow rapidly and after 30 days they measure 800-1000µm in the length and have begun to coil inside the cell. The capsule finally measures 0.4 – 0.6 by 0.25 mm at about three months; calcification begins after six to nine months but the larvae in them may live for several years. Cases in which the larvae lived of 11 and even 24 years have been recorded. In the cysts the larvae can't develop further but must await ingestion of the infected meat by another host. In this other host the larvae are liberated from their cysts in the stomach and grow to adults in the intestine, beginning to deposit larvae within six to seven days. Prenatal infection with this parasite appears to be rare, but it had been produced experimentally following heavy infections.

VI. Epidemiology:

Independent sylvatic and synanthrofic zoonotic cycles of infection occur. The sylvatic cycle involves wild carnivores such as jackals, will boars, black bears, bush pigs etc. and these animals maintain the transmission. However, many may become infected following the ingestion of meats from wild boar, heal, walrus etc. Trichinella of man associated with work prepared meat for exotic dishes. The synanthrofic Zoonotic cycle occurs primarily in swine and rats; occasionally cats, dogs and man may become infected. Out brakes of Trichinellosies have been associated with horses. Some offered to be due to contamination of horse meat with pork, but in addition, horses are susceptible to infection and *T. spiralis* and may be infected if processes horse feed contain remnants of infected meat.

VII. Pathogenesis and clinical signs:

The parasite is of principal importance in human medicine and it is unusual for any obvious clinical entity to be associated with the infection in domestic / wild animals. The intestinal form may produce a certain amount of irritation and cause a marked interior heavy infection. The most important pathogenic effects are produced by the larvae in the muscles. Heavy infections may lead to death, especially through paralysis of the respiratory muscles. The clinical signs which accompany trichinosis are very variable and may simulate those of variety of other diseases; they include diarrhea, fever, retroperitoneal pain, stiffness and pain in the affected muscles, dyspnoea, hoarseness, sometime an edema of the face and deafness. A marked eosinophilia is usually present. A crisis is usually reached after about four week when the egg production of the females begins to decline and the larvae become encapsulated.

Epidemics of Trichinellosies occasionally occur in human beings when a number of people eat insufficiently cooked Trichinellosies meat of a pig.

VIII. Diagnosis:

A correct diagnosis can only be achieved by demonstrating the trichinella larvae in the muscle obtained either from biopsy or autopsy. The following measures may be adopted.

i.   Stool examination for adult worms or for larvae (rarely recovered)

ii. Blood examination shows cosinopritic leucocytosis / eosinophilic 15-50%)

iii. Sereological tests, such as compolement fixation procipicin and bentonite flocculation test.

iv. Muscle biopsy: The excised tissue may be pressed flat between glass slides and examined under the low power of microscope.

v.   Skin test: Intradermal injection of 0.1 ml of 1 n 10,000 dilution of the antigen causes as immediate erythematous patch. A +ve test persists for 10-20 years.

vi. X-ray examination may be of value if the cysts are calcified, but the worms are too small to be detected on an x-ray plate.

IX. Treatment:

Promising results have been obtained in the treatment of trichinosis by thiabendazole. Corticosteroids have been found to be helpful in alleviating clinical symptoms.

X. Prophylaxis

The measurements include

i. Careful inspection of meat at slaughter house and
ii. Avoidance of eating raw or imperfectly cooked pig's flesh.

XI. Control and Prevention:

Human Trichinellosies is disseminated chiefly by the pig. This animal is most usually infected for raw garbage which contains scraps of trichinous eats. Grain fed pigs usually shows a low incidence of infection. However, prohibition, on the feeding of garbage regulations requiring garbage to be cooked before being fed to pigs contributes to reducing the incidence of swine Trichinellosies.

Man usually acquires the infection mainly from pork / partly cooked. Prophylaxis should therefore aim at the elimination of uncooked garbage in the feed of pigs and as for as man is concerned. The thorough cooking of all pork products and the meat of child animals such as wild boar, fox, bear, walrus, etc.

XII. Pathogenicity:

Mode of infection is by ingestion of infected pigs' flesh, raw or insufficiently cooked food containing the viable larvae.

The symptoms are grouped as follows

a. Stage of intestinal invasion (incubation): This is the period (5-7 days) during which larvae grows into adult worm and the of begins to discharge larvae into the circulation the symptoms are chiefly gastro intestinal.

b. Stage of larvae migration: The invasion of muscles occurs from the 7th to the 10th after infection. The manifestations are remittent temperature, certicanil rash, and sublingual "splinter hemorrhage: edema of the cycloids and myositis. There may be respiratory symptoms, myocardiitis and protease neurological signs imitated by invading larvae. At this stage there may be profound and at time fatal toxemia.

c. Stage of encystment: This occurs only in striated muscles while in other tissues they degenerate and are absorbed. The symptoms may clear up rapidly or disappear gradually as the larvae become encysted or may larvae permanent injury.

II. Necator americanus

Phylum:	Nematoda
Class:	Secernentea
Order:	Strongylida
Family:	Ancylostomatidae
Genus:	*Necator*
Species:	*americanus*

I. Introduction: (Common name: American hookworm)

Hook worm disease in man is caused by two different worms, *Necator americanus* or the new world hook worm and *Encylostoma duodenal* or the old world hook worm. The two species of adult worm can be readily differentiated but their ova.

II. Geographical distribution:

It is the most common species in Srilanka and India (Except in Punjab and U.P). Although first discovered in America, it is more likely of African origin. From its original focus (Tropical and South Africa) it has spread to India, Far East, Australia and America.

III. Life cycle:

Adult hook worms are about 6-12 mm long and live firmly attached by their mouth parts to the mucosal wall of the human small intestine from which they such the blood.

The fertilized of hookworm produces fertile eggs almost continuously at the rate 10,000-25,000/day. These are passed which the host faeces. In soil, that is in moist and warm the eggs hatch in a day or two inter motile, non-infective rhabidiform larvae.

For the next 5 days these feed, grow and develop in the soil, finally elevating into long slender, non-feeding filariform larvae which are infective for man.

Presented with human epidermis the larvae penetrate it by mechanical and lytic action; eventually reacting through blood stream by which route they proceed to the lung capillaries into the alveolus spaces. They make their way up the bronchi and trachea to the pharynx then are swallowed. The life span of an adult hookworm is usually 1-2 years rarely 6-5 years.

IV. Pathogenesis and disease characteristics:

There is an important differentiation between hook worm infection and hookworm disease.

Hookworm infection indicates that the organisms have entered and are multiplying in the host, number of worms present. Hook worm infection includes only few worms that the host has no symptoms. At the other end, when hundreds of worms larvae puncture the skin, skin irritation percussive edema and erythematic occur at this penetration site.

Larvae passing through the lung may produce lesions in heavy infections. Many migrating larvae damage may be too extensive that it results in pulmonary disease.

Hundreds of hook worm in a single host may cause anemia, enteritis, abdominal pain and diarrhea. In severe infection the anemia is believed to cause of a myocardiitis and cardio enlargement which may be fatal.

And one adult hookworm may move around in its feeding and is responsible for numerous minute bleeding ulcers. Relation exists between hookworm disease and the host's nutritional state. Hookworm disease is rare when nutrition is good. Several hookworm diseases occur in those places where malnutrition is found.

V. Epidemiology:

Hook worm parasite infects hundreds of millions of people. Necator tends to occur more in tropical areas. Ancylostoma in subtropical areas. Their distribution is governed by both their moisture and temperature requirement in the soil and by the habits of their human hosts. Larvae develop best at temperature between 23-30C is constantly moist soil.

Chances of continuing the cycle are greatest where human excrete is placed directly on the soil and where people go bare foot.

VI. Diagnosis

    i.   Hook worm infection is generally diagnosed by binding the thin shelled colorless eggs in the patient's faeces. In a heavy infection they may be numerous as to be fund on direct microscopic examination of faecal smear. In human infections egg may be found only in stool specimen.

ii.   From a therapeutic stand point it may be important for the physician to know which hook worm species is causing the patient infection. Hook worm species differentiation can be made, however on the basis of morphological differentiate in the adult worms. In initial case of anti hookworm therapy will yield adult worm that can be identified, then the most effective therapy can be instituted.

iii. It is helpful in diagnosing disease such not merely to know that the patient is infected but how heavily he is infected. There are standard ways to do this. They are based on determining the number of eggs per gram of the patients focus several determination over a number of days yield more reliable results than a single determination knowing.

   a.   About how many eggs of hookworm produce in a day
   b.   The daily output of faeces per day and
   c.   The number of eggs per gram of faeces.

It is relatively easy to calculate the approximate number of worms present. Diagnosis of the disease cannot be made on the basis of the clinical picture.

VII. Treatment:

Patients which human hookworm infection lacking symptoms or anemia need not be treated. Often are treated with a single oral dose of tetrachorethylene.

VIII. Prevention and control:

Hookworm infection is limited by attacking that part of the worm's cycle outside of man. This includes prevention of soil contamination by sanitary disposal of human excretes and prevention of new infection by wearing of shoes. Educating the public may also help. Additionally in areas where infection is heavily endemic, drug treatment of the population at range may reduce hookworm (disease) incidence.

III. *Ancyclostoma duodenale*

Phylum: Nematoda
Class: Secernentea
Order: Strongylida
Family: Ancylostomatidae
Genus: *Ancylostoma*
Species: **A. duodenale**

(Common name: The Old World Hook Worm)

I. Introduction:

The parasite was first discovered in 1838 by an Italian physician Angelo Dubini. The pathogenesis and mode of entrance of the larvae into man was worked out by Loss in 1898.

II. Geographical distribution:

It is widely distributed in all tropical and subtropical counties, occurring in places wherever humidity and temperature are favorable for the development of larvae in the soil. It is found in Europe, North Africa (Prevalent in Egypt) Indian, Srilanka, Central and North China, Pacific Islands and Southern States of America.

III. Habitat:

The adult worm lives in the small intestine of man, particularly in the jejunum, less often in the duodenum and rarely in the ileum.

IV. Morphology:

Adult worm: It is small, grayish white, cylindrical worm, when freshly passed it is reddish brown in color due to the ingested blood in it intestinal tract. The anterior end is bent dorsally (backward), hence the name hook worm. The oral aperture is not terminal but directed towards the dorsal surfaces. The large and copious buccal capsule is provided which 6 teeth, 4 hooks like on the ventral surface of 2 knobs - like triangular plates on the dorsal surface. There are five glands connected which the digestive system; oesophageal glands, secretes a ferment which prevents the clotting of blood.

The sexes are easily differentiated by their size and shape of the tail and the position of the genital opening. The worm assumes y shaped figure during copulation.

Copulatory Bursa: This consists of 13 lobes: 1 dorsal and 2 lateral; each lobe is supported by chitinous rays; the dorsal lobe contains 3; the two lateral lobes contains 1o rays; total number of rays are 13.

Male and female:

Male:

   i.   Size: Smaller about 8 mm in length
   ii. Posterior end: Expanded in an umbrella like fashion
   iii. Genital opening: Posterior opens which the cloaca.

Female:

    i.   Size: Longer than male with about 12.5 mm in length
    ii.   Posterior end: Tapering, no expanded bursa.
    iii. Genital opening: At the junction of posterior and middle third of the body.

V. Life cycle:

The life span of the adult worm in the human intestine has been estimated to be about 3 to 4 years.

Eggs: The eggs are passed out which the faeces and the distinctive features of the egg are as follows:

    i.   Oval or elliptical in shape measuring 65 μm in lengths by 40μm in breath.
    ii.   Colorless
    iii. Surrounded by a transparent hyaline shell – membrane
    iv. Contains a segmented ovum usually which 4 blastomas; has a clear space between the egg shell and the segmented ovum.
    v.   Flats in saturated solution of common salts.

The eggs, when passed out with the faces, are not infective to man.

No intermediate host is required like other helminthes, multiplication of worms does not occur inside the human body. Man is the only definitive host for *A. duodenale*. The following are the various stages of the life cycle.

Stage 1: Passage of eggs from the infected host: The eggs containing segmented ova with four blastomas are passed out in the faces of the human host.

Stage 2: Development in soil: From each egg a rhabidiform larvae hatches out in the soil in about 48 hours. The rhabidiform larva moults twice, on the third and 5th day. It then develops into filariform larva, the infective stage of the parasite. The time taken for the development from eggs to filariform is an average of 8 to 10 days.

Stage 3: Entrance into a new host: the filariform larvae are infective to man. The larvae cost off their sheaths and gain entrance to the body by penetrating the skin.

Stage 4: Migration: On reaching the subcutaneous tissue the larvae enter into the lymphatic or small venues, and are carried via the right bent into the pulmonary capillaries; where they break through the capillary walls and enter into the alveolar spaces. They than migrate on the bronchi, trachea and larynx. Entering the oesophagus, a third moulting takes place and a terminal buccal capsule is formed, migration is about 10 days.

Stage 5: Localization and laying of eggs: the growing larvae settle down in the small intestine, undergo 4th moulting and develop into adolescent worms. In 3-4 weeks time, they are sexually mature and the fertilized eggs are passed in the faces, the cycle in thus repeated. The interval between the time of skin infection and the first appearance of eggs in the faeces, is about 6 weeks.

VII. Pathogenicity and Clinical Features:

The worm causes hook worm disease or encyclostomasis in man, characterized chiefly by anemia.

Mode of infection: This occurs when man walks bare foot on the faeces contaminated soil. The filariform larvae penetrate directly and their entry sites are:

   i.   The thin skin between the toes.
   ii.   The dorsum of the feet and
   iii. The inner side of the soles.

In case of gardeners and minors, the skin of the hands may be the portal of entry. Infection may also occur by the accidental drinking of water contaminated with filariform larvae.

1. Pathogenic effects caused by Encylostoma larvae.

   a.   Lesions in the skin:
        i.   Encylostoma dermatitis or ground itch occurs at the site of entry.
        ii.   Creeping eruption is a condition in which the filariform larvae wander about the skin in an aimless manner producing a reddish itchy papule along the path traced by the larvae.

b. Lesions in the lungs: Bronchitis and bronchi, pneumonia may occur when the larvae break through the pulmonary capillaries and enter alveolar space. A marked eosinophilia occurs at this stage.

2. Pathogenic effects caused by Adult worms:

The adult worm inhabits the small intestine attaching them to the mucous membrane by means of buccal armature. A severe progressive anemia of microcystic hypochronic type develops.

Immunology: the endemic areas most patients have minimal intestine infection and number of significant symptoms of anemia and this may be attributed to the development of a partial immunity. A heavy infection with symptoms of anemia may result from the failure of development of immunity.

Causes of anemia:

1. Chronic blood loss: This results from the which drawl of blood by
    a. Parasites for their food and
    b. Chronic hemorrhages from the punctured sites. The loss of hemoglobin for each 12 worms to be 1%.
2. Nutritional defects: Some other contributory factors include deficiency of the available iron and other haemopoietic substances in the diet. Thus depending upon the nature of the nutritional defect, the type of anemia may vary with iron deficiency,

a hypochronic microcystic anemia and with deficiency of both iron and vitamin B12 or folic acid causes dimorphic anemia.

Clinical features of hook worm anemia:

i.   Gastro – intestinal manifestations: These may be dyspeptic troubles associated with epigastric tenderness stimulating duodenal ulcers.

ii. Patient may have abnormal appetite showing prevented taste for such things as earth, mud.

iii. Bowels are generally constipated.

Effect of anemia:

i.   The skin assumes a sallow appearance and the mucous membrane of the eyes, lips and tongue shows extreme pallor.

ii. The face appears puffy which the swelling of lower eyelids and then is edema of the fact and ankle.

iii. The general appearance of the patient is a plumpy individual with protuberant abdomen and dry lusterless hair.

iv. Growth and development in children may be retarded.

VIII. Morbid anatomy:

1.   Intestinal lesions by adult worm: Areas of small extravasations of blood, some fresh and some old; the latter indicated by pigmentation. If the examination is made which in 3 hours after death,

the worms may still be attached to the centre in the mucosa. If the examination is delayed, the worms are free in the human bowel.

2. Effects of anemia: Fat changes in the liver and heart may between well marked in severe cases. Bone marrow often shows an erythroblastic reaction and the yellow marrow is transformed into a red formative marrow.

IX. Diagnosis:

1. Direct Method:
   i. Examination of stools: A macroscopic examination of stools is necessary to find the adult worms which may be passed out spontaneously or after a vermifuge.
   ii. Study of duodenal contact: the materials obtained by duodenal incubation may sometimes reveal either eggs or adults worms.

2. Indirect Method:
   i. Examination of blood: This is carried out to ascertain the nature of anemia and the presence of eosinophilia.
   ii. General examination of stools: In majority of cases, hook worm anemia, test for occult blood in the stool gives a +ve reaction. Charcot – Leyden crystals are often found in the stool

X. Treatment: For the treatment of hook worm infection the following steps are to be taken

a) Expulsion of worms by anthelmintic and
b) Treatment of anemia

Specific anthelmintic treatment should not be started if the hemoglobin is below 30%. In such case, anemia is to be treated first with iron and after the hemoglobin level is above 50% specific antihelmantic is to be administered.

For hookworm infection the antihelmantic drugs used are tetrachorethylene, bephomium hydroxymaphthoate (more effective against a – duodenale).

Hookworm anemia responds readily to oral iron (Ferrous sulphate 200 or 400 mg thrice daily, according to the tolerance of the patient). Folic acid and vitamin B12 may be indicated in some cases.

X. Prophylaxis: The following measures may be adopted:

1. Attack on adult parasite: treatment of carriers and diseased person simultaneously which whole sale treatment of community.
2. Attack on larvae: Prevention of soil – pollution by proper control of sewage disposal. Disinfection of faces or soil
3. Personal protection: Wearing of boots and gloves.

UNIT I – V

PATHOGENIC TREMATODES

I. Fasciola hepatica

Phylum:	Platyhelminthes
Class:	Trematoda
Subclass:	Digenea
Order:	Echinostomida
Suborder:	Echinostomata
Family:	Fasciolidae
Genus:	*Fasciola*

Species: *hepatica*

I. Introduction:

Fasciola hepatica is a common parasite of sheep, cattle, goats, deer and other herbivorous animals. The common name of *F. hepatica* is the sheep liver flack, the common live fluke. Amongst the Trematodes, this was the first to be discovered by Jehan de Bric in 1979. These are endoparasite in the liver and bile duct of sheep; goat; cattle even human being is also affected.

The disease caused by the fluke is referred to as "Liver rot". Man is an accidental host. *F. hepatic* is the main species which causes human fasciloiasis throughout the world.

II. Geographical distribution: (Cosmopolitan)

Fasciola hepaticas is World Wide in distribution particularly sheep and cattle raising areas are the primary zones where human being are also infected. Its other Indian species *F. gigantic* (=indica) is found in the bile of buffalo cow, goats and pigs.

III. Morphology:

Adult worm: It is a large leaf – shaped fluke, measuring 3cms in length by 1.5cm in breadth and brown to pale grey in color. There are two suckers. The anterior end bearing the oral sucker forms a conical projection. The posterior end is rounded. The acetabulum is situated in a line with the projection posterior. The genital system opens on the ventral surface near the acetabulum. Life span of the adult worm in sheep is 5 years and in man is 9 to 13 years.

Eggs: the characteristics of eggs are as follows

1. Large, operculated, avoid in shape, brownish yellow in color.
2. Size 140 μm by 30 μm.
3. Contains a large unsegmented ovum in a mass of yolk cells.
4. Excreted with the bile into the duodenum and then passed out along with the faeces.
5. Can develop only in water.

IV. Life cycle:

F. hepatica passes its life cycle in two differentiate hosts:

Definitive host: Sheep, goat, cattle or man. Adult worm is present in the liver. Reservoir host is primarily the sheep.

Intermediate host: Snails of the genus *Symnaea* larval development proceeds in this snail.

The eggs passed out in the faces of definitive host, mature in water; inside each egg a citied miracidum is developed in the course of 2 to 3 weeks time. On escaping from the egg the miracidum finds its way to its suitably intermediate host. Inside the lymph spaces of the molluscan host, the miracidum passes through the stages of sporocyst, two generations of radial and finally to the stage of cercariae. The whole cycle take a period of 30 to 60 days. The mature Cercariae escape from the snail into the water and encyst in blades of or water. The encysted cercariae are swallowed along with the grass or water crest by herbivorous animals (their final hosts) and occasionally by man. On entering the digestive tract the metacercariae excyst in the duodenum migrate through the intestinal wall into the peritoneal cavity, penetrate the capsule of the liver, traverse its parenchyma and ultimately settle in the biliary passages and taking about a month to migrate and grow to sexual maturity. The eggs are liberated in the faeces through the bile in about 3 to 4 months after infection. The cycle is then repeated.

V. Pathogenicity:

Human infection is not exceptional and the symptoms of fasciloiasis include biliary colic with persistent vomiting, diarrhea and tender hepatomegaly with peripheral eosinophilia (40-85%). It is most common in sheep and cattle raising counties.

F. hepatica is primary responsible for producing a disease in the animals, known as "liver rot". During migration of the young worms, they cause extensive damage to the liver tissue and in heavy infections, may lead to portal cirrhosis, while in the biliary passages, they may interfere with normal flow of bile, causing obstructive jaundice. The mature worms cause marked pathological changes in the biliary tract by mechanical irritation as well as by their toxic secretion. The biliary epithelium proliferates, giving rise to adenomata.

VI. Diagnosis: This is based on the finding of eggs in stool or in bile obtained by duodenal incubation. The eggs of *F. hepatica* and *F. buski* are indistinguishable. For immunodiagnostic antigen from adult worm is used for complement fixation test and skin test.

FASCIOLA BUSKI

Phylum:	Platyhelminthes
Class:	Trematoda
Subclass:	Digenea
Order:	Echinostomida
Suborder:	Echinostomata
Family:	Fasciolidae
Genus:	*Fasciolops*
Species:	*buski*

I. Introduction

Fasciola buski is commonly known as intestinal fluke. It is the largest trematode infecting man. It was first described by Buski in 1843 in the duodenum of an East Indian sailor who solid in London. It is a parasite of man and pig.

II. Geographical distribution:

It is an Asiatic trematode and has been reported from China, Thailand and Malaysia, in India – Bengal, Assam and other oriental regions.

III. Habitat:

The adult worm lies in the small intestine of man and pig. The normal host is the pig which serves as the reservoir of infection for man.

IV. Morphology:

Adult worm: It is the largest trematode parasiting man and measures 2-7 cm in length, 8-20mm in breadth and 0.5 - 3mm in thickness. It is elongated and oval in shape, the anterior being narrower than the posterior. The acetabulum is large and lies close to the oral sucker. The two intestinal caeca don't bear any lateral branches. The genital system follows the same general pattern of Trematodes. Life span of the adult worm is short (not more than 6 months).

Eggs:

1. Large operculated, avoid in shape, brownish yellow in color.
2. Size 140μm by 30μm.
3. Contains a large unsegmented ovum in a mass of yolk cells.
4. Exerted with the bile into the duodenum and then posted out along with the faces.
5. Does not float in saturated solution of common salt
6. Can develop only in water

V. Life Cycle:

Fasciolopis buski passes its life cycle in two different hosts:

Definitive hosts: Man and pig, adult worms are found in small intestine.

Intermediate host: small flatly coiled aquatic snails of the genus Segmentina.

The eggs are passed out in the feces of definitive hosts, mature in water. Inside each egg a ciliated miracidum is developed in the course of 2-3 weeks time. On escaping from the egg the miracidum finds its way to its suitably intermediate host. Inside the lymph spaces of the molluscan host, the miracidum passes through the stages of sporocyst. Two generations of radiae and finally to the stage of cercariae. The whole cycle takes a period of 30-60 days.

The cercariae, on coming out of the snail, encysts on fresh water plants, especially side pools of water, caltrop, the bulb of water chestnut and other aquatic vegetation which are fertilized with moist soil and grown in shallow ponds where the snail abound. On being swallowed, the metacercariae excyst in the duodenum and the liberated young worm attach themselves to the intestine wall developing into adult worms in about 3 months time. The eggs are then liberated and the cycle is repeated.

VI. Pathogenicity:

Mode of infection: eating infected plants or raw food studs (peeling it with the teeth)

Portal of entry: alimentary canal.

Infecting agent: excysted cercariae (metacercariae)

Site of localization: small intestine (duodenum and jejunum)

Infection with Fasciolopsis buski is known as Fasciolopsiasis. The disease is characterized by asthenia, mild anemia and chronic diarrhea. In heavy infections, anemia becomes more intense and absorption of by-products of the worm leads to edemas and eosinophilia.

VII. Diagnosis:

This is based on the history of residence in endemic areas and on the findings of eggs in stool by microscopic examination. The eggs of F. buski and F. hepatica are indistinguishable. Adult worms may be recovered after a purgative or an anthelmintic.

VIII. Treatment: specific anthelmintic drug includes tetrachorethylene.

IX. Prophylaxis: this consists of the following:

   i)   Sterilization of the night-soil before being used as a fertilizer.
   ii) Destruction of molluscan hosts by Copper sulphate solution (1 in 50000 strength) and
   iii) Avoid eating raw vegetables (water caltrop and water-chestnut) or before consumption they should be cooked or immersed in boiling water for few minutes.

Schistosoma haematobium

Phylum: Platyhelminthes

Class: Trematoda

Subclass: Digenea

Order: Prosostomata

Family: Schistosomatoidea

Genus: *Schistosoma*

Species: *haematobium*

I. Introduction:

This vesicle blood fluke, formerly known as Bilhar Zia haematobium has been endemic in the Nile valley in Egypt for millennia. Its eggs have been found in the renal pelvic of an Egyptian mummy dating from 1250-1000 BC. The adult worm was described in 1851 by Bilharz in Cairo. The life cycle, including the larval stage in the snail was worked out by Feiper in 1951 in Egypt.

II. Geographical distribution:

Various parts of Africa and Middle East. Gadgil and Shah in 1952 reported a few cases from India (Ratnagiri in Maharashtra state).

III. Habitat:

Adult worms live in copula, pelvic venous plexus-vesicle, prostatic and uterine plexuses of veins.

IV. Morphology:

The adult worms live in the vesicle and pelvic plexus of veins. The male is 10-15mm long by 1mm thick and covered by cuticle of finely tuberculated. It has two muscular suckers, the oral sucker being small and the ventral sucker large and prominent. The adult female is long and slender. 20mm by 0.25mm with the cuticle tubercles confined to the two ends. Life span is 20-30 years.

V. Life Cycle:

S. haematobium passes its life cycle in two hosts:

Definitive host: Man, adult worm living in vesicle and prostatic venous plexus.

Intermediate host: Fresh-water snail.

The embryonated eggs are passed with the urine of the definitive host and gain access to water. Miracidum hatched out of the eggs; move freely in water in search of their intermediate host snail. The miracidum is transformed into a tubular sporocyst; later multiplies and forms a second generation of sporocyst. Several weeks after the infection, where no further multiplication occurs, the daughter sporocyst gives rise to larval forms, cercariae which are infective to man. The cercariae break off from the sporocyst and escape from the snail into water.

Infection results when human beings bath in the infected water, the cercariae penetrates through the unbroken skin directly. On entry the cercariae cast off their tail and gets access to a peripheral venule. From here they are carried through the right heart into the pulmonary capillaries. It requires some days for the larvae to pass through the capillary bed in the lungs and they are carried through the left heart into the systemic circulation. Now they gain access to mesenteric artery, pass through the capillary bed in the intestine and enter portal circulation (taking 5 days to reach the liver). After sexual differentiation, they move out of the liver against blood current, migrating into the inferior mesenteric vein, rectal venous plexus, pelvic veins and eventually enter the vesical plexus of veins (take 1 – 3 months time). When the worms are sexually mature they copulate and the fertilized females lay eggs which are ultimately voided with the urine. The cycle is thus repeated.

VI. Pathogenicity:

An individual bathing in an infected pool or comes in contact with contaminated water is liable to be infected. The cercariae stick to the surface of the skin of the swimmer or bather, by means of their ventral suckers (acetabula) and as the water begins to evaporate, penetrate the skin.

Infecting agent: Cercariae – these have a free swimming existence and can live in this state for a maximum period of 3 days.

Portal of entry: skin

Site of localization: vesical plexus of veins (urinary bladder).

Pathogenesis: the terminal spined eggs may erode blood vessels and cause hemorrhages. Eggs get deposited in the tissue, act like foreign protein and have an irritative effect leading to round cell infiltration and connective tissue hyperplasia. The tissue reaction in these cases produces what is known as formation of a "pseudo tubercle" around each egg. Large and progressive granulomas are found only around the calcified eggs and may cause a diffuse fibrosis.

VII. Clinical features:

The disease caused is referred as Schistosomiasis haematobia. Evolution of the disease passes through three phases:

i) By the cercariae at the site of entrance: this is particularly seen with the cercariae of non-human (adult worms in birds or small mammals) local reaction.

ii) By the toxic metabolites liberated during the growth in the portal blood of the liver: general reaction characterized by fever, urticaria, and eosinophilic leucocytosis, enlarged tender liver and palpable spleen. The symptoms appear between the 4th and 5th week of the infection.

iii) At the time of laying eggs: this may be regarded as a localizing symptom, generally occurring within 3 – 9 months of the infection. The characteristic manifestation is a painless terminal haematuria (at first by the reversible granulomatous inflammatory reaction to eggs and later by the irreversible fibrosis and calcification).

VIII. Diagnosis:

This is based on the demonstration of eggs in:

a) a microscopic examination of urine (centrifuged deposits)
b) a piece of vesical mucosa removed by cystoscopic biopsy. The excised tissue is divided into two pieces. One is compressed between two slides and examined for eggs under the low power of microscope. The other piece is placed in a fixative for histological examination.

Other tests include:

i) Blood examination: Eosinophilic count, aldehyde test (often +) or complement fixation test-sera of patient (reacts + with cercariae antigen obtained from infected snails liver).
ii) Intradermal skin test with cercarial antigen: immunological tests are group specific and give positive results.

IX. Treatment:

The drugs having specific actions are nitrothiazole compound, niridazole, nilodin, hycanthone, trivalent antimony compounds such as tartar emetic, fovadin, anthiomaline, antimony dimercaptossuccimate.

XI. Prophylaxis:

The preventive measures include:

i)   Eradication of the disease in man
ii)   Prevention of pollution of water with human excreta
iii)   Destruction of the snail vector in endemic areas and
iv)   Avoidance of swimming, bathing, wading or washing in infected water.

UNIT VI

PATHOGENIC CESTODES

ECHINOCOCCUS GRANULOSUS

Phylum: Platyhelminthes
Class: Cestoda
Order: Cyclophyllidea
Family: Taeniidae
Genus: *Echinococcus*
Species: *granulosus*

I Introduction

Tape worms belonging to the genus Echinococcus have their definitive host, a carnivore's predator that preys on the intermediate host which is usually a herbivorous mammal. The domesticated example of this Echinococcus granulosus: the dog tape worm or the hydatid worm, which has the dog as the definitive host and sheep and man as the principal intermediate host. In man it causes unilocular echinococcosis or hydatid disease.

The adult worm was discovered by Hartmann (1695) and the larval form by Goeze (1782)

II. Geographical distribution:

Although the hydatid disease is worldwide in distribution, it is commonly found in those countries where sheep and cattle raising constitute an important industry and consequently there is a close association between man, sheep and dog. It is more a disease of temperate climates than of tropical areas.

III. Habitat:

Man harbors the larval form and not the adult worm which is however found in the small intestine of dog and other canines.

IV. Morphology:

Adult worm: it is a small tapeworm, measuring 3-6mm in length. It comprises of a scolex (head) neck and strobila consisting of 3 segments. The first segment is immature, the second one is mature and the last one is gravid. The terminal segment is biggest measuring 2-3mm in length by 0.6mm in breadth. The scolex bears four suckers and a protrusible rostellum with two circular rows of hooks. The neck is short and thick.

Egg: it is ovoid in shape and resembles other eggs of Taenia. It measures 32-36μm in length by 25-32 μm in breadth and contains a hexacanth embryo with 3 pairs of hooks. The egg is infective to man, cattle, sheep and other herbivorous animals.

Larval form: this is found within the hydatid cyst developing inside the intermediate hosts. It represents the structure of the future of the scolex. On entering the definitive host, the scolex with the four suckers and rostellar hooklets, becomes evaginated and develops into an adult worm.

V. Life Cycle:

The worm passes the life cycle in two hosts:

i)   Definitive host: Dog, Wolf, Fox and Jackal. The adult worm lives in the small intestine of these animals that discharge a large number of eggs in their faces. The dog is the optimum definitive host.

ii)   Intermediate host: Sheep, pig cattle, horse, goat and man. The larval stage is passed in these animals and man, giving rise to hydatid cyst. The sheep appears to be the optimum intermediate host.

The eggs are discharged with the faces of the definitive host. These are swallowed by the intermediate host, while grazing in the field, and also by man (particularly children) due to intimate handling of infected dogs. In the duodenum, the hexacanth embryos are hatched out. After 8 hours after ingestion, the embryos bore their way through intestinal wall and enter the radicals of the portal vein. The embryos are carried to the liver and arrested in the sinusoidal capillaries. Some of the embryos pass through the hepatic capillaries enter the pulmonary circulation and filter out in the lungs (liver acts as the first filter and lungs acts as the second filter). Practically all the organs of the domestic animals may be invaded but they are chiefly found in the liver and lungs.

Wherever the embryos settle they form a hydatid cyst, the young larva. A hydatid cyst developing from a single egg may contain 1000's of scolius. A fully developed scolex is an end product and its presence inside the hydatid cyst is a sign of a "complete biological development". These fertile hydatid when ingested by the dog, are capable of growing into adult worms in about 6-7 weeks time in the intestine. Thus the cycle is repeated.

As the dogs have no access to the hydatid cyst developed in the viscera of man, the life cycle of the parasite comes to a dead end. The natural cycle is thus maintained by dog and sheep.

VI Pathogenicity:

The adult worms in dogs do not cause much inconvenience. The larval worms in man cause unilocular hydatid disease.

Mode of infection: the eggs in the dog's faces are ingested by man by means of direct contact with infected dogs, by allowing the dog to feed from the same diet or by taking uncooked vegetables contaminated with infected canine faces.

Infecting agents: eggs in dog's faces.

Portal of entry: Alimentary tract.

Sites of localization: viscera / liver, lungs and other organs. Infection is generally acquired in childhood though the disease does not become manifest before adult life.

VII. Clinical features:

The clinical manifestations are entirely dependent upon local signs and if the cyst is situated superficially, it may cause a visible swelling. In majority of cases the disease remains latent for many years and its presence is only detected by autopsy or by its pressure effects on the surrounding tissues or when the cyst ruptures. The pressure symptoms will vary according to the site of the cyst. Rupture of a hydatid cyst is associated with anaphylactic symptoms and formation of localized or generalized secondary echinococcosis.

VIII. Laboratory diagnosis:

This consists of the following:

i)   Casoni's reaction: an immediate hypersensitivity skin tests introduced by Casoni in 1911. Intra dermal injection of 0.2ml of a fresh sterile hydatid fluid produces a large wheel which multiple pseudopodia; it fades in an hour. Hydatid fluid from human cases or from animals is used as antigen.

ii) Blood examination: a generalized eosinophilia of 20-25%

iii) Serological test: this is carried out with hydatid antigen (fluid) found to be positive.

iv) Haemoagglutination test: using fresh or formalinised sheep red cells sensitized with tannic acid coated with Echinococcus antigen.

v)   Radiological tests: this is often helpful in the diagnosis of hydatid cyst of lungs and liver. Owing to the saline contents, the cyst is relatively opaque and costs a characteristic circular shadow with a sharp outline. In case where the long bones are involved a mottled appearance is seen.

IX Treatment:

There is no specific drug. Treatment for infection is surgical excision and even this procedure is often unsuccessful of impractical.

X. Prophylaxis:

This consists of the following

    i)   Prevention of infection of dogs and the deworming of dogs in endemic areas and

    ii)   Personal prophylaxis (cleaning of hands before eating). Laboratory workers should guard against contamination of fingers while examining dog's faces.

HYMENOLEPIS NANA

Phylum: Platyhelminthes
Class: Cestoda
Order: Cyclophyllidea
Family: Hymenolepididae
Genus: *Hymenolepis*
Species: *nana*

I Introduction

It is commonly known as the dwarf tapeworm. Hymenolepis nana is the smallest and the commonest tapeworm found in the human intestine. The Hymenolepis refers to the thin membrane covering and nana from nanus meaning dwarf. It is cosmopolitan in distribution but is more common in the warm than in cold climates. It completes its life cycle in a single host.

II Geographical distribution:

Cosmopolitan in distribution, but it is more common in the warm than in cold climate.

III Habitat:

The abode of the adult worm is the small intestine of man. It is also found in rodents, especially in mice and rats.

IV Morphology:

Adult worm: it is the one of the small intestine Cestodes infecting man. It is small and thread like measuring 1-4cm in length and a minimum diameter of 1mm. Life span of the adult worm is short (about 2 weeks)

The Scolex: it is globular, has four suckers and is provided with a short retractile rostellum armed with a single row of hooklets numbering 20-30. The neck is long.

Proglottides: the number of segments is about 200. Genital pores are marginal and are situated on the same side. The uterus is transverse sac with a globulated wall while there are three testes.

Eggs: these are liberated in the faces by gradual disintegrate of the terminal segments. The characteristics of the eggs are as follows:

   i)   Spherical or oval in shape measuring 30-45mm in diameter
   ii) There are two distinct membranes: outer membrane is thin and colorless and the inner embryophore encloses an oncosphere with 3 pairs of lancet shaped hooklets.
   iii) The space between two membranes is filled with yolk granules and polar filaments emanating from little knobs at either end of embryophore.

V Life cycle:

No intermediate host is required and the entire development from the larval to the adult stage takes place in one host. With the ingestion of a fully embryonated egg, a hexacanth embryo is liberated. It burrows into the villi of the anterior part of the small intestine and develops in about 4 days time to a typical larval stage called "cysticercoids". After reaching maturity, the villus ruptures and the larva (scolex) re-enters the lumen of the small intestine. Later it attaches to another villus further down and in the course of a fortnight develops into a adult worm, strobilisation is rapid and in about 30 days after the infection, the eggs begin to appear in the faces. Some of the eggs remaining in the bowel can start the cycle over again.

Besides the direct cycle referred above, an indirect cycle has been demonstrated. Certain rat fleas and beetle act as intermediate host and transmit marine infection to man.

VI Pathogenicity:

Mode of infection: first infection occurs through ingestion of food contaminated with eggs liberated along with the faces of an infected man or rodents. Afterwards autoinfection increases the number of parasites. There are usually no symptoms but with heavy infections there is abdominal pain and diarrhea.

VII Diagnosis:

This is based on the finding of characteristic eggs in a microscopic examination of a sample of faces.

VIII Treatment:

It is not easy to dislodge by same drugs as used for other tapeworm infections. Praziquantel and nicbramide are effective in treatment.

IX Control:

Prevention is by proper personal hygiene.

DIPHYLOBOTHIUM LATUM

Phylum: Platyhelminthes

Class: Cestoda

Subclass: Eucestoda

Order: Pseudophyllidea

Family: Diphyllobothriidae

Genus: *Diphyllobothrium*

Species: *latum*

I Introduction:

It is commonly known as the fish tapeworm or the broad tapeworm. Infection with this tapeworm is called diphyllobothriasis. The head of the worm was found by Bonnet as early as 1777 but it was only in 1917 that its life cycle was worked out by Janicki and Rosen.

II Geographical distribution:

It occurs in central and northern Europe, particularly in the Scandinavian countries. It is also found in Siberia, Japan, North America and Central Africa. It has not been reported in India.

III Habitat:

Adult worm lives in the small intestine (ileum) of man, dog cat, fox and other fish eating mammals.

IV Morphology:

The adult worm is yellowish-grey in color with dark central markings caused by the egg-filled uterus. It measures 3-10 meters in length. An individual worm may live for a period of 5-13 years.

The scolex is elongated and spoon shaped and measures 2-3mm in length by 1mm in breadth. It bears two slit like grooves situated on the dorsal and ventral surfaces respectively. There are no rostellum and no hooklets. The neck is thin and unsegmented and is much longer than the head.

Proglottides: these are 3000 – 4000 in number. The segments are greater in breadth than in length. A mature segment is practically filled with male and female reproductive organs. The terminal segments are apt to be shrunken and empty owing to the constant discharge of eggs through the uterine pore. Later the dried up segments break off and are passed in the host's faces. There are three genital pores. The ovary is bilobed, the uterus is large and remains coiled in the form of rosette.

Eggs: these are passed out in the host's faces. The characteristic of the eggs are as follows:

- i)   Oval and brown in colored
- ii)   Contains abundant of yolk granules and an unsegemented ovum.
- iii)   There is an inconspicuous operculum at one end with a small knob at the other end.

iv) Does not float in saturated solution of common salt. The eggs are not infective to man.

Larval stages: these are passed first in water and then in the respective intermediate hosts. There are three stages of larval development. The first stage larva is known as Coracidium which develops from egg in water. The second stage larva is known as Procercoid and is found inside the Cyclops, the first intermediate host and the third stage larva is known as Plerocercold and is found in a fresh water fish, the second intermediate host. Single egg gives rise to single larva.

V Life Cycle:

Definitive host: man, dog and cat. Man is the optimum host. The adult worms are found in the small intestine.

Intermediate host: aquatic animals where the larval stages are passed –

a. The first intermediate host is a fresh water crustacean, a Cyclops or a diaptomus
b. The second intermediate host is a fresh water fish, pike.

Development of egg in water and liberation of a ceracidium: the operculated eggs are liberated through the faces of definitive hosts in water. Three pairs of hooklets called ceracidium develop within the egg shell in 2 week. This larva is ingested by the Cyclops.

Larval development inside Cyclops: inside the intestine of Cyclops, the larva penetrates, through the intestinal wall and comes to rest inside its body cavity. In about 3 weeks an elongated solid body with a caudal spherical appendage containing the six known as procercoid larva. Developing larvae is in turn enters the second intermediate host, a fresh water fish.

Larval development inside fish: in the intestine of fish, the procercoid larva after freeing itself, passes through the gut wall and rests into the liver muscles in the mesentery and proceeds to develop further. In 1-3 weeks, the procercoid larva changes into a "sparganum" or "plerocercoid" larva. The larva is marked by irregular unsegmented wrinkle. The smaller bodies lie straight in the flesh but the larger ones remain bent and twisted.

Infection of man and development of adult worm: the plerocercoid larva is infective to man. It is not destroyed by ordinary salting or smoking and therefore with eating of these insufficiently cooked fish or raw fish man is infected. Inside the intestine of man the larva develops into an adult worm and starts discharging eggs which are passed along with the faces. The cycle is then repeated.

VI Pathogenicity:

Mode of infection: by ingestion of imperfectly cooked infected fish or roe containing plerocercoid larvae. The symptoms are gastrointestinal disturbance and anemia.

VII Diagnosis:

This is established by a microscopically examination of faces for the characteristic operculated eggs. Segments passed with the faces may be recognized by the character of the uterus and the position of the genital pores.

VIII Treatment:

Specific antihelminties are mepacrine, dichlorophenol and nichoamide

IX Prophylaxis:

Preventive measure includes prevention of pollution of water, efficient disposal of sewage, personal prophylaxis in endemic areas. Consume thoroughly cooked fish.

About the Author

The author Dr. K. Renuka born and brought up at Gulbarga, Karnataka India did her P. G. from Department of Zoology, Gulbarga University, Gulbarga securing three Gold medals and was on top in merit list of P G students. She completed her Ph. D. with Merit fellowship awarded by Gulbarga University, Gulbarga. She is working as Guest Lecturer in Department of Zoology, Gulbarga University, Gulbarga. She has published research papers in international peer reviewed journals and still continues her passion for research.

Printed in the United States
By Bookmasters